FIRST AID HANDBOOK

BRANDA NURT

Table of Contents

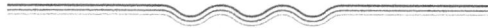

First Aid Handbook
How to Heal from Wilderness Accidents

First Aid Handbook
How to Heal from Urban Accidents

First Aid Handbook
How to Heal from Domestic Accidents

FIRST AID HANDBOOK

How to Heal from Wilderness Accidents

BRANDA NURT

Introduction

Few people are truly prepared to handle the likely accidents that can happen in the wilderness. Whether you're out hunting, hiking, fishing, or camping, you need to be prepared. This book can not only prepare you to have proper emergency plans in place but can and should serve as an emergency reference if you have an injury that happens out in the wilderness. Injuries that happened in the wild do not have the benefit of immediate professional medical attention, and very few are prepared and confident to handle the extent of some of these injuries.

Don't get confused about what to do, or what should happen next. Instead, go through this book, find the injury that you're facing and learn what to do. Have a complete list of what you should do, what you should not do, and how to assess the injury's seriousness. This book was written to be a complete guide to help people in emergencies address minor to severe injuries in the wild.

Chapter 1

Prepare and Plan

Outdoor sports and activities are resurging across the nation. More people are returning to classic sports such as hunting, fishing, and finding more enjoyment in camping when they have during the initial boom of the tech revolution. Many of us had lost touch with the outdoors, but if you're someone who has newly rekindled their love of getting out into nature or has spent years pursuing this passion, then you know you can never be too prepared.

The modern-day masters of the wilderness may very well be the Boy Scouts. Back in the early 1900's Baden-Powell put together a Scouting for Boys pamphlet, and shortly after, the Boy Scouts of America was founded. One of the overarching elements that come out in not only the Boy Scouts of America but all other variations of them across the world is to be prepared. This phrase of "be prepared" should be familiar to anyone who spends a reasonable amount of time outdoors, especially if they're away from immediate medical care. If you know that you're going to be generally far away from medical facilities, then it's best to take up the Boy Scouts' mantle and focus on being prepared. Because of the high interest in wilderness recreation, more and more people are experiencing outdoor injuries and even outdoor illness. There are serious repercussions for not being prepared in these situations.

Unfortunately, not everyone can foresee the worst-case scenarios. In fact, if you're planning a fun camping trip, then the first aid kit might be the last thing on your mind. This chapter will briefly cover how you could prepare and how you'll need to plan if the preparations weren't complete.

Before Every Wilderness Excursion, Do These Things

With well-known survival stories such as 127 Hours, wilderness excursions often call for a set approach. There are a few things you should always do before you leave your home and go into the wild or outdoors, even if you are with people.

Always:

- Let people know when you are leaving and when you plan to return.

- Let someone know whether you will, or will not, have cell service. If you don't know, assume not.

- Inform someone of where you will be or a roundabout region.

- Tell someone your plans, are you hiking, fishing, climbing, or camping? This can help in emergency response situations.

- Never:

- Assume that someone will find a note that you left with the above-listed information.

- Assume that someone will know you went out for the weekend/week.

- Give inconclusive dates for your return.

There are far too many stories of people being lost for days or weeks because they didn't convey information to someone who could have gotten them help. In some of these situations, many people involved have experienced severe injuries, including weather-related injuries that could have resulted in a fatality. It may seem like common sense, but always give the information above to someone that you know would take immediate action if you didn't arrive home on time or keep up communication as planned.

Preparation is key in handling any wilderness injury. It's often a substantial-quality to have if you're going to be an outdoors person, and if you are new to outdoor sports, then it's something you should begin practicing immediately. There is no way to overvalue preparation.

A Quick Guide on First Aid Kits

Many people do have first aid kits on hand when wilderness injuries happen. You're very standard, off-the-shelf, first aid kit should include gauze pads, antiseptic spray, antibiotic cream or gel, gloves, adhesive bandages, scissors, and adhesive or medical tape. Things kits will not address all of the most common outdoor injuries. Still, they do provide valuable resources that can come into play to treat almost any injury you may experience in the outdoors. These kits can be valuable, but you can build your kit or purchase a hiker's kit to have a wider variety of resources and tools to use in the event of an emergency injury.

What do you need in a first aid kit?

- Alcohol/hydrogen peroxide
- Athletic tape or wrap
- Band-aids
- Burn cream or spray
- Cold/hot packs
- Compass
- Flashlight
- Gauze
- Insect repellent
- Medical tape
- Mouth barrier for CPR
- Pain reliever/fever reduce such as Tylenol
- Pocket knife/Swiss Army knife
- Safety pins
- SAM splint for immobilization
- Scissors

- Swabs

- Syringe

- Tweezers

- Waterproof matches

A first aid kit with all of the items listed above will prepare you to handle not only cuts and scrapes but also to fight off infection, splint sprained or broken bones, give CPR, treat burns, address head injuries, and more.

In addition to everything listed above, you may pack your own personal prescriptions, hydrocortisone cream, antihistamines for treating allergies, aloe vera, and more. It is possible to get all of these things packed together in a small travel case or travel bag. You don't need a completely separate backpack to hold all of these items, as most are extremely small, and most manufacturers of high-end first aid kits know that size is an issue for hikers and campers.

You can easily find premade first aid kits in most stores that have a pharmacy or online. Additionally, sports stores such as Big 5 or Dick's Sporting Goods, and local sporting goods stores will often have specialized first aid kits for hikers, camping, and even fishing. These kits will often have specialized tools or materials to help handle the most common injuries associated with that outdoor sport. You can also build your own first aid kit, and if you do this, then you'll know that everything in the kit was put in with a specified purpose and that you know exactly what is in the kit.

That brings us to another common issue, not knowing what is in your first aid kit or how to use the materials. If you purchase a first aid kit, go through it thoroughly and evaluate each item's use or purpose. Items that are marked with their prescription name or scientific name are things you can research ahead of time and then write in a Sharpie across the packaging the intended use or household name. For example, if something is marked antihistamine, you might write with a marker "allergy treatment." Other common items include Polysporin, which is an antibacterial gel, and Hydrocortisone, or corticosteroids cream for rashes and skin irritants.

If you have other people going with you regularly, such as a family camping trip, go through the materials with key people you would expect to jump into action in the event of an injury. Some people attempt to go through an entire kit with children, that is entirely up to you. Most often, the best you can expect from children, especially small children, is the application of ice packs and Band-Aids. Make sure that everyone on a camping trip knows where to find a ranger station or how to contact someone who can reach help, whether through satellite phone, cell phone, which may not have service, and how to find a nearby payphone. Going into the woods, going camping, heading into the wilderness for a hike, and any other outdoor sport can be extremely enjoyable and rewarding. But it is important to prepare for the possible worst-case scenarios.

If You Are Caught Unprepared, Do These Things
If you do not have a first aid kit, you need to assess your resources immediately, and likely evacuate. If you are hiking or fishing and

sustain any type of injury without having a first aid kit, it's best to call it a day and go home. If you are out camping, or in a national park, you should locate the nearest Ranger Station to get medical supplies.

Being caught unprepared happens. It's important that you don't panic because it's in moments of panic that things go wrong. If you have a cut, scrape, or sprain, you can likely treat the injury with materials you're wearing or what you have on hand just in basic camping supplies.

Realizing that you're unprepared after an injury is always disheartening, and I can put a damper on the entire situation even with the injury in mind. However, it's critical to realize that being unprepared for an injury in the wild happens more often than any experience outdoors person would like to admit.

Each section of this book will include a shortlist of emergency resources that you may have on hand, even if you don't have a first aid kit. Injuries in the outdoors call for people to be extremely resourceful. You'll often surprise yourself with how quickly you can devise a plan and a calm and decisive action even when you don't have an elaborate first aid kit.

In the Event of Every Injury

There are some things that everyone should do when faced with any type of injury, at home or the outdoors. These steps will help ensure that the person giving treatment has the patient's best interest in mind. The person injured may not be able to respond appropriately or fully grasp the gravity of the situation. When people are hurt, they may go into shock, they may become hysterical, and it's important that anyone around them fully assess the circumstances.

Make a Plan

The very first thing you should do after an injury is to make a plan. Have a plan of how you will approach treating the injury and assessing the extent of the damage. This may happen in a matter of seconds. You may even immediately know that the injury needs to be cleaned, kept dry, and wrapped. That is a plan.

However, when faced with less common injuries such as burns, you may not know what to do. That is where guides like this come into play. Your initial plan may be to reference the emergency injury guide and determine exactly how you will need to treat it. Plans are important, whether you're prepared or not.

Keep a Level Head

Take a second and take a deep breath. Someone with shaky hands and is in a moment of panic or is a little scatterbrained can do more damage than if the injury waits a moment for treatment. A level head is absolutely critical, improperly treating injuries. It can be a very scary moment, but in these instances, trust treatment to the calmest person.

One thing that helps in getting a level head in intense or high anxiety situations is to step away momentarily. Take one or two steps away and take a deep breath. Think aloud and express what you intend to do or what you think the best plan is out loud.

Set Clear Milestones to Determine If A Situation Is Getting Better or Worse

Every type of injury can range from very minor to deadly. You will need to determine exactly where on the scale of seriousness of the injury falls, and how to monitor whether the injury is getting better or worse.

As part of the segmented approach to this book, there are clear milestones listed under each section to determine how serious an injury is and if after treatment the injury is improving or if the person's health is deteriorating. Evaluating milestones that you set will largely depend on observation. Proper observation involves not only watching the wound or the injury, but also the person. Any change in behavior, appearance, or bodily response, such as a fever, can signify that someone is improving or getting much worse.

Often, there are evidently good and bad changes to any type of injury. If you notice any bowel or off smells, evacuate immediately because it's likely the onset of early infection. This is common among burns, flesh wounds, and more. Additionally, if someone is entirely unresponsive or is becoming disoriented, then evacuate immediately.

Know-How to Get Medical Attention

There are certainly some situations where the injured person genuinely no opportunity has to receive professional medical attention. However, many people who are in state or national parks do have access to medical attention. Knowing where your local ranger station is, or how to find a nearby medical center can drastically change the outcome of a wilderness injury.

Often Park Rangers are available at the end of trails, and on some trails or frequented areas of the parks, there may be landlines that connect directly to nearby ranger stations. Additionally, you may be able to obtain medical attention through your phone if you have service. If you do not have service, you may start evaluating other means of emergency medical attention such as flares, hazard lights, and even sending a person out to find help and return with assistance.

Evacuation

Throughout this book, you'll see the term evacuate, or evacuation. This means leaving your current area. Of course, the intent in doing this is to seek immediate medical attention from a professional. People often don't want to call it quits on their camping or hiking trip because someone burned their palm or twisted their ankle. This isn't unreasonable.

Many people have carefully thought out their plans for hiking, camping, fishing, outdoor sports, and excursions into the wilderness. However, there are times when you need to immediately start making your way back to civilization for medical treatment. If you know that without a doubt you are at least 24 hours away from the nearest town or city that would have a medical center, then some injuries may call for evacuation even when they seem mild, or the patient seems completely fine. For example, near-drowning victims will often report being absolutely fine as soon as they are breathing and rest a bit. However, there is a slim chance of dry drowning, or secondary drowning, which can happen between one and 48 hours after the drowning incident. If secondary drowning were to occur, say six hours or 12 hours after the incident, and you are 24 hours away from the nearest medical center. You must begin moving towards civilization immediately after the event.

Always use your best judgment when planning to evacuate, if you know that you were only a short way away from a nearby medical center, then there may be no need to brush off. When deciding whether or not to evacuate, give careful consideration to how far away you are from nearby medical professionals and whether you have easy communication with emergency services.

What You Can Expect from This Book

Throughout this book, you can expect to receive full guidance for each type of common wilderness injury. That includes a list of how to assess the seriousness of the injury, determine if it requires emergency medical intervention, and how to treat it.

Each section will also include a guide on what not to do; many common-sense steps in treating wounds can do more damage. You will learn how to respond in emergencies and what actions to take in which order.

It is important to address that we are not responsible for the improper application of procedures or techniques. It is always best that people go through formal training for medical procedures and techniques before spending a substantial amount of time outdoors. If you have time to prepare, look at your local CPR and first aid certification options. For advanced certification, you can evaluate the options for a Red Cross certification. While in life-threatening situations, immediate action is often necessary, improper action can also lead to harm. We are not responsible for the harm that happened from improper or incomplete use of any medical procedure or medical technique.

Chapter 2

Cuts, Scrapes, and Abrasions

Cuts and scrapes are among the most common injuries in the wilderness and households as well. Cuts and scrapes are easy to evaluate and diagnose, but many are not familiar with the full extent of serious injuries involving cuts, or possible penetration. These injuries often happen off the trail, or deep in the backwoods.

Campers often experience these as they may fall, scramble, or injure themselves while setting up equipment. Hikers often experience these when they fall or stumble and may impale or cut themselves on natural elements such as branches, bushes, or rocks. Fishers, come with a variety of different issues when regarding cuts, and abrasions. They may have hurt themselves on a hook, injured themselves on equipment or items within the boat or the deck, or may sustain serious injuries in the water. No matter how the cut, scrape, abrasion, or impalement happened, you'll need to treat the wounds the same.

Flesh wounds all call for the same method of treatment, but the big issue that people come across is understanding how the injury happened and how severe it is. Your injury may have been preventable, and being aware of it can help your group avoid it. Additionally, understanding the injury's extent can change how quickly you respond to the accident and how much effort you put into your aftercare. For example, a small scrape might be something you slap a Band-Aid on and call it a day, whereas a deep puncture wound would need periodic cleaning and bandage changes every few hours.

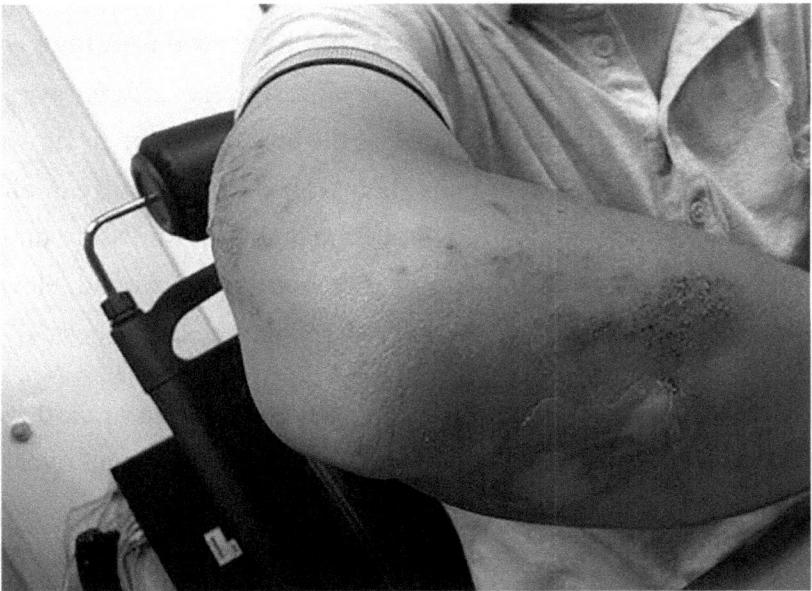

Flesh Wounds Can Happen Anywhere

Flesh wounds really can happen anywhere, and they are so common that the entirety of a basic first aid kit is meant to address cuts and scrapes. The commonality of flesh wounds has often left people severely underestimated the need for immediate medical attention. Many people who experienced flesh wounds and had complications later remarked that they thought the wound was fine.

When last untreated, flesh wounds can fester, which can lead to infection, and even the need to amputate the limb. You must take immediate and decisive action with flesh wounds. The good news is that there is one set regimen for treating flesh wounds regardless of the seriousness. We will discuss the seriousness of flesh wounds later and how to determine if you need to take immediate action to get to professional medical help, or not.

Slow, Clean, Bandage, Moisturize and Keep the Bandage Dry

There's a simple approach to handling almost every different type of flesh wound. First, you'll want to slow the bleeding. Turn to slow the bleeding of a cut, scrape, or piercing injury, use clean gauze or cloth to cover the injury, and place a moderate amount of pressure on the wound. While covering and applying pressure to the wound, elevate the moon, preferably above the injured person's heart or chest.

This accomplishes a few things. First, the clean gauze or cloth will give the blood something to adhere to, so it's not running all over the place. Second, the pressure will help the soft tissue damage begin recovery. Finally, elevating the wound will help slow the blood flow to that area, reducing the amount of bleeding.

After you have substantially slowed if not stopped the bleeding, then you can begin cleaning the wound. This might seem counterintuitive, but you don't want to start cleaning the world while blood is still free-flowing.

When cleaning the wound, you will want to use two primary tools. First, you will need to use sterilized tweezers to remove any large pieces of debris. You can sterilize plastic tweezers with rubbing alcohol or hydrogen peroxide, and you can sterilize metal tweezers either with rubbing alcohol or heat from a flame. After you use tweezers to remove large debris, you will need to use water or a sterile alternative.

Do not clean a wound with found water, or even spring water. Even when the water looks like it runs clear, it can contain life-threatening bacteria. Instead, use drinking water that you brought with you to clean the wound. If you do not have clean water to spare to clean the wound, you may use rubbing alcohol or hydrogen peroxide if you have liquid forms. When cleaning a wound with water or a sanitary alternative, you will want to get pressure behind that fluid. EMT Personnel tends to prefer to use a plastic syringe when cleaning a wound, because of the pressure and force that it comes with. If you have a plastic syringe in your first aid kit, use that to clean the wound. However, you can also accomplish a fair amount of water pressure by puncturing the lid to a water bottle and squeezing the water bottle or squeezing a water sack and pinching the nozzle, so it creates one steady stream.

It was widely accepted that dry wounds were least susceptible to bacteria. However, the medical community has since proven that open wounds need to stay moist but not necessarily wet. Before you wrap the wound, cover the wound and antibiotic gel such as Neosporin or petroleum jellies such as Vaseline or Aquaphor.

When the wound is clean, you can bandage it. Ideally, the bandage will be comfortable sitting, but not so tight that it cuts off circulation.

Most people tend to wrap bandages tightly and sure that the bandage is comfortable and doesn't move. A bandage will likely involve multiple layers. If the cut is generally clean, you will want to use adhesive strips to create a butterfly closure. If the cut is jagged or a puncture wound, then you'll want to cover the wound and wrap around that entirely.

While you wanted to moisturize the wound itself, you don't want the dressing to get wet. Keeps the dressings dry for as long as possible. Initially, you will want to check the wound about 30 minutes after you dress it, and a few hours after that first checkup. Afterward, you will want to change the dressing every 12 hours regardless of how clean it looks.

What to do when you aren't prepared:

If you did not have a first aid kit on hand, then you probably don't have gauze or anything to sterilize tweezers with, you probably don't have tweezers, and you may not have the adhesive tape or bandages necessary to wrap the wound securely.

To start, gather whatever potable water you have or begin boiling natural water to clean the wound. You will still want to elevate the wound and use a clean cloth to cover it to slow the bleeding. Then clean the wound and dress it with the cleanest material you have available. It is critical that the wound not remain open to the elements.

Depending on the severity of the cut, you may need to call it quits and evacuate the patient immediately. If the cut seems minor, then head to a nearby ranger station to get proper medical supplies to wrap and protect the wound.

How to Determine if this is an Emergency

What is the difference between a minor cut, and something that needs medical attention right away? The first thing to assess is the depth and length of the cut or abrasion. If the cut is more than half an inch long, then it is likely that the cut needs stitches and that it needs stitches soon. Additionally, if the cut is so deep that you cannot hold the edges together with only a slight amount of pressure, then the person may need emergency medical attention.

Now, the other element to consider when determining if this is an emergency or not is the amount of bleeding. If the wound continues bleeding after about five or 10 minutes of direct pressure and elevation, then they likely need emergency medical assistance, and you need to evacuate immediately. Additionally, if the wound is spurting blood or it is coming out in rhythmic gushes, then you may have severed something rather important. You could likely lose a substantial amount of blood in a small amount of time. If blood is spurting or gushing, then evacuate immediately and seek immediate and professional medical attention.

You may notice immediate signs of healing, but not seeing me find does not inherently mean that the situation is more urgent than you initially believed. For example, a cut involving a flap of the skin may begin healing in the course of a few hours. You may notice that the skin is staying in place, or that a scab is forming because the blood has thickened. In contrast, a puncture wound may be an entirely different matter. Puncture wounds may take up to two days to show early signs of healing, and it may take two weeks or longer for puncture wounds to heal even when they didn't need stitches. Don't use the visual determination for a healing timeline to decide that the injury is less or more severe. If anything, use visual signs to detect possible infection and determine whether or not you may need additional medical help in treating the wound.

What to Do with Flesh Wounds

We've covered a few elements of what to do already, but here is a quick list of exactly what you should do in response to any type of flesh wound.

1. Elevate the wound

2. Apply pressure using a clean cloth or gauze

3. Wait for bleeding to slow, if bleeding does not slow or stop after five or 10 minutes, seek immediate medical attention.

4. Clean the wound with potable water. If drinking water is not available, you may use alcohol or hydrogen peroxide.

5. Put Neosporin, Aquaphor, Vaseline, or similar over the wound.

6. Attempt to use adhesive strips to close or completely cover the wound.

7. Bandage the wound over the adhesive strips in a comfortable fit.

8. Keep bandages dry.

Additional tips to keep in mind:

- Always wear gloves if they are available, whether you're treating yourself or someone else.

- Monitor the wound closely for the first 30 minutes.

- Check the circulation, motion, and sensation of the body part with the wound.

- If bleeding is severe, use a tourniquet. A tourniquet is a strip of fabric or other material used to temporarily decrease blood flow to the area if it should help slow or stop the bleeding.

- If the wound comes from a bite, evacuate immediately, and seek professional help.

- If possible, avoid using alcohol or hydrogen peroxide as they can damage healthy tissue.

Many of these tips are meant to protect the person with the injury and the person treating them. Even if you are treating yourself, doing things like wearing gloves can change whether you get an infection or not. The bacteria, germs, and oils on your hands can affect an open wound. In that same thought process, it's always better to cover a wound than to let it be open. Many people have grown up with the idea of saying, "let the wound breathe," and that's terrible advice, especially in the backwoods. Bacteria and germs are all around us, and if you're cut in your home, then most of those present elements are familiar to your body. Even familiar bacteria can be very dangerous and lead to infection, but in the wild where nearly everything is foreign, you run even bigger risks. It is better to cover the wound with a clean shirt, towel, or blanket than it is to leave the wound open to the elements.

Additionally, you may need to keep the severity of the wound in mind during treatment. If a wound is very severe and you are evacuating to seek professional medical treatment, it may be best to use a tourniquet to decrease blood flow and slow the bleeding.

Using a Tourniquet

When using a tourniquet, you will want to tie the fabric or constricting device at least five cm or about two inches above the open wound. Additionally, you'll want to tie it around an area of the limb that has one bone. For example, tying a tourniquet around the upper portion of the arm rather than over the forearm. The latter has two bones connecting the wrist to the elbow. Ideally, a tourniquet should be closer to the trunk of the body.

After tying the tourniquet around the limb, you'll want to place a knife, pair of scissors, or other sturdy and straight objects directly over your knot. Then tie a knot over that object and twist it to tighten the tourniquet. This is known as a windlass, and you can secure the wind last after tightening it by tying another knot to prevent the windlass from unwinding.

Tourniquets should only be used in extreme situations, as a last resort for major, uncontrolled bleeding.

What Not to Do with Flesh Wounds

The list of things not to do has a couple of surprises. Often, we are taught basic first aid that drastically differs from recommended first aid.

Do Not:

- Attempt to clean a very deep wound, as it will cause more blood loss.

- Assume that a wound is clean; even if you can't see debris, clean it.

- Remove a stuck object.

- Push any body parts "back" into place.

- Allow the wound to "air out."

Other common things that you should avoid doing if at all possible, include using strong antiseptics. Many people grew up believing that you needed to apply iodine, rubbing alcohol, or hydrogen peroxide to open wounds. While these are good disinfectants and are certainly excellent options for cleaning utensils such as tweezers or scissors in first aid kits, they shouldn't be used on open wounds. The only time that they should be used on open wounds as when potable water is not available. This is one primary difference between treating a flesh wound and treating burn wounds; those that involve punctures or cuts can withstand some damage from these harsh antiseptics if it's absolutely necessary. Burn wounds cannot take this damage. If you are treating a flesh wound associated with a burn, then turn to

Chapter Five for full instructions on treating flesh wounds related to burns.

Aftercare

Aftercare for a flesh wound generally calls for carefully watching the wound for infection. If the wound came from an animal or rusty metal, you might need to seek medical attention as soon as possible to get treatment for possible diseases carried by animals or tetanus.

Signs of infection of a flesh wound include redness around the wound, red streaks spreading from the wound, extreme tenderness and swelling, yellow or green colored pus, drainage from the wound, and fever. Infection is treatable, but this is not something you can treat in the wild, you do need to see a doctor and get the appropriate antibiotics for the infection.

If you don't experience any signs of infection, then it is likely that you can continue to redress the wound and wash it gently, and it should heal on its own. If you need stitches, see a doctor as soon as possible, so they have a fresh wound to work with. Additionally, a few days of healing may help a doctor determine whether or not stitches are necessary if it seems like your injury is on the cusp of possibly needing stitches.

Flesh wounds are the most common injury in the wilderness and when camping, closely followed by sprains and burns. However, flesh wounds can vary drastically. A deep puncture wound may be a greater cause for concern than a long-running scratch. The elements to always keep in mind are the size and depth of the wound. Never underestimate the ability of a flesh wound to become very serious in a short time frame as an infection is not only possible but, in the wilderness, likely. Additionally, you might take greater care on your next excursion to pack a fully planned out first-aid kit.

Chapter 3

Sprains and Strains

A sprain is a common injury that happens when the ligaments or the fibers connect one bone to another, either stretch or tear. Sprains usually happen when you twist an ankle or overextend your shoulder. While you might think this is a very mild injury, injury to ligaments can be very serious. They're also generally uncomfortable, and in the way of first aid, there's not usually much you can do.

If you believe that you or someone you're traveling with has experienced a sprain, then make sure to follow the RICE method for treatment. The good news is, you have about all the equipment necessary to diagnose a sprained, and often doctors that do diagnosis sprain simply end up with this diagnosis because they've ruled out all other more serious injuries.

Similar to sprained is a strain. A strain happens when a tendon is stretched or pulled away from the bone and can range from mild to quite serious. The tendon itself is the strip of fibrous material that connects the end of a muscle to the bone. It is the reason why your muscles can flex and respond in normal ways. Strains are seen less frequently in the outdoors because they often happen over a long duration of time. You may strain a tendon through years of sports or overexerting yourself physically.

Common Muscle Injuries and Sprains

Sprained ankles, twisted knees, banged up shoulders, and whiplash is among the most common sprains and soft-tissue injuries. The general recommendation is that anyone who can't put weight on the injured joint should seek medical attention. That's often not necessary, as most adults don't go to their physician for a sprained ankle. However, it's likely that if your injury happened outdoors, it might be more serious. Unlike trying to catch yourself after tripping on a curb or a stair, it is more likely that twisting or spraining your ankle in the outdoors was more strenuous.

Common signs of a sprained include pain or swelling, difficulty using or flexing the joint, and bruising, or even warmed in the injured area. Most strains or sprains can heal on their own in a two to three-week window, and there's very little that doctors can do. In fact, the course of treatment often involves reducing pain and ensuring that the soft tissue of the joint does not incur further injury.

RICE: Rest, Ice, Compress, Elevate

The rice method is pretty straightforward, and it's a common treatment for a wide variety of soft tissue damage. But, there's a right way to perform these steps and a wrong way. Many people don't realize that administering the RICE approach can go wrong, cause more pain, or even cause more injury to the joint.

Rest

The very first step is to rest the joint. You're going to continue resting, by avoiding any activities that cause pain, or discomfort. Additionally, if you noticed some activities cause the swelling to increase, it's best to avoid those as well. Now, where this goes wrong is that you should avoid all physical activity. There is a stark difference between resting the joint and not doing anything. You do want to keep moving around, but you also don't want to take the "walk it off approach." The best thing to do in most situations with sprains is to allow the insured person to rest and use their gauge to determine which activities cause pain or discomfort.

One of the excellent things about the RICE treatment is that it doesn't use any resources for a first aid kit. And you don't run the risk of infection or exposure to bacteria that you do with open wounds. This step and RICE call for no resources, which means you can do it with or without a first aid kit.

Ice

Now there is a right way to ice an injury. You don't want to simply throw a cold pack on there and leave it on until the patient complains. Cycling ice or cold treatment is the best approach. Use an ice pack from a first aid kit or the coldest water that you can find and treat the injured area for 15 to 20 minutes. After 15 or 20 minutes, give the injured area a break from the cold treatment, and restart another 15 or 20 minutes of cold treatment every two or three hours for the first few days following the injury.

The coldest water available might be the water in your ice chest that is mostly ice. That is perfectly fine to use. The coldest water available might be a running spring nearby, and that is perfectly acceptable. The only element here that you need to worry about is the coldness of the water. Unlike open wounds, there's no need to use only potable water or ice.

It is always ideal to have ice packs on hand, but many people find themselves out in the woods without ice packs or crack packs that cool after a disruptive action such as cracking or shaking them. If you have a sprain or strain and know that you'll be needing an ice pack every few hours, you can make your own ice pack from items you have in your first aid kit or items you have around the camp or in your pack. You can, of course, simply freeze water in a plastic bag. However, for longer-lasting ice packs, mix one part of rubbing alcohol to three parts of water in a plastic zip-top bag. Suck out as much air as possible and leave the bag and an ice chest or very cold running water for a few hours.

Salt is another good alternative if you're trying to make ice packs on-site. What salt does is lower the freezing temperature of the water, and it makes the pack slushy rather than watery. Add about two tablespoons of salt for two cups of water in a zip-top bag and place it in an ice chest, or cold running water. If you don't have an ice chest, for example, if you were out hiking and weren't planning on camping, then you can often use running spring water, or cold natural water to help bring the temperature of the solution down. Aside from having something to season your food with it, this is a great reason always to carry salt in your pack.

Compression

After the first cold treatment, you'll want to apply a firm bandage, preferably elastic, to help contain the swelling. Many people in the outdoors have found that a combination of a stretch or elastic bandage and non-stretch bandage works best. There is also a right and a wrong way to apply bandages, and doing so the wrong way can decrease circulation, eliminate sensation in the area, and even result in blistering and skin damage.

When compressing a sprain, start wrapping with an elastic bandage from the edge of the joint farthest from the heart. In most cases, with an ankle, you're going to be starting at the bottom of the ankle. Then, about halfway up the joint, switch to a non-stretch bandage, or greatly reduce the amount of stretching or pulling that you're applying to the bandage as you are wrapping. Some people recommend wrapping at the digits closest, especially if the injured joint is a wrist or an ankle. That's not always necessary, but it can be good practice.

If you do not have bandages or wraps, then it is possible to begin compression with clothing material. It is not ideal, often clothing material especially meant for athletic wear or outdoor wear, will stretch too much to compress the injury properly. However, you may use a combination of a cloth material and manual compression to help contain the initial swelling. If you don't have bandages to address the joint injury right away, then it may be best to evacuate.

Elevation

You want to elevate the injured area of the body above the chest. The full combination of the rice treatment often ends up with the injured person lying down or reclining so that the injured joint can be elevated, and you ensure that they're generally resting the joint. Elevating the injury above the chest does help reduce the blood flow, which can slow down swelling in the joint. This approach also helps gravity reduce the swelling, and less swelling often means less pain for the patient.

How to Determine if this is an Emergency

Sprains are hardly ever an emergency, and strains are only emergencies in unique situations. Of course, it is possible to experience a severe soft tissue injury, such as detaching a muscle or completely detaching ligament connections. These are also rather unlikely.

However, some people do confuse a sprain with a broken bone or a severely damaged joint. If you're diagnosing the injury, then you will want to emphasize the range of mobility and level of pain.

The first question is, can the person move the joint on their own? This bit of the test will likely be painful, but it is necessary.

The second question to evaluate whether this is possibly a more serious injury is to determine if the joint looks normal. A sprain may come with swelling and even some unexpected bumps, but if anything seems to be completely out of place, then it's likely something is broken.

The final later determination when assessing whether or not this is an emergency is to check in on the injury after RICE treatment. After a few rotations with cold treatment, so maybe eight to 12 hours after the initial injury, if you see continued swelling, broken skin from swelling, extensive bruising, or if the pain has gotten worse, then you likely need to arrange for medical treatment. In the event of the symptoms listed above, you may be dealing with ligament or muscle detachment rather than a mild soft tissue injury.

What to Do with Sprains and Strains

Of course, there are a few things that you should do with sprains, and the first may actually cause pain to the injured person. If you are treating yourself, this may be slightly easier to handle. You will need to rotate the foot, wrist, shoulder, or injured joint to determine a specific point of tenderness and the range of motion. Doing this will help you splint or wrap it in a way that is comfortable and reduces pain.

It is typically best to try to immobilize the joint completely, but that's not always possible. Immobilizing the joint with a compression bandage should not completely restrict movement but should instead limit the range of motion.

If the injured person still seems able to walk freely, then simply tape the ankle and splint it around their shoe.

The best way to splint a sprain is with a c-splint. A c-splint will cradle and support the joint across its flat most point and then wrap around the ankle. For example, with a sprained ankle, you would place the initial wrapping across the bottom of the heel, then fold each end across the top of the ankle and wrap behind the back of the ankle. Alternatively, you can use the strip pattern, which calls for the use of adhesive tape, creating a stirrup shape around the injured joint.

Eventually, you will want to arrange for medical attention. Sprains often don't call for an emergency room visit, and if you show up to the emergency room with a mild sprain, they will likely send you home. Instead, when you do get back home or back to civilization, arrange for a standard doctor's appointment with a general practitioner. There's no need to go to an emergency room or an urgent care center unless you suspect that the injury may be more serious than a sprain.

If you suspect that you have a strain, rather than a sprain, make sure you express that concern to your doctor. Depending on the extent of the strain, surgery may be needed, or they may suggest a more intensive course of physical therapy.

What Not to Do with Sprains

This is one of the few injuries in the wilderness that actually doesn't call for immediate evacuation. If you are out camping or fishing, then wrap the sprained joint elevated, undergo the RICE treatment, and continue with your plans if it won't cause further injury. There is very little that doctors can do, and even diagnostic testing such as x-ray, MRI, CT scans, or even an ultrasound won't produce conclusive results. Now, if you think that the bone or joint might be broken in some way, then evacuate and seek medical attention.

The most common thing that people do with sprained that they should not do is heat treatment. You do not need to rotate a cold and a hot pack or cold and hot treatment for the injury. The issue in this particular situation with heat treatment is that swelling occurs because of bleeding into the tissue, drawing more blood to that specific area. Using a heating pad or a hot towel can increase swelling drastically.

The final issue people fall into with treating a sprain or a strain is telling the injured person to walk it off. Walking it off does not work; it causes more damage to the joint and can cause lasting damage to the soft tissue. Now, a few days after the injury, you can begin to put some weight or cautiously use the joint. Rest on that first day or so is very important.

Aftercare

Standard aftercare instructions for a sprain often include seeking Physical Therapy. Although this is likely a mild soft tissue injury, it can be painful, and it can lead to long-term pain or even long-term injury if it doesn't receive proper treatment. As you treated the wound in the outdoors, then it's likely that you didn't take the exact actions that a doctor might have. When you're done with your time in the wilderness, then contact your local doctor and explain to them what happened and what steps were taken to treat the injury. They may keep an eye on it, they may send you home with at-home physical therapy exercises for the joint, or they may refer you to a local physical therapy center.

In addition to physical therapy, the doctor may provide you with a breeze on the splint or cast so that the joint can have set restrictions in movement. These support devices not only reduce pain but can also help the injury heal by eliminating unintentional stress or strain.

One rather important thing to note is that once you have sprained a joint, that joint is then more likely to undergo sprains in the future. The muscle may have healed to the best of its ability, but one sprain will often lead to another on the same joint. Strains will often happen the same way as well. If you have previously sprained an ankle, or if this is your first sprain, then you should consider adding compression wraps or garments to your first aid kit. Someone who knows that sprains are not only possible but likely should carry compression garments so that the compression applied to the injury is steady and consistent. It is easier to slip on a compression wrist sleeve than it is to tightly and accurately wrap a sprained wrist or elbow joint. Always look at any injury you experienced in the wilderness as an opportunity to better prepare yourself next time by adding items to your first-aid kit.

Chapter 4

Near Drowning

Near drowning can be rather common when people are fishing, boating, or camping near a lake or river. It hardly ever comes from outright complacency, because most people don't know the real signs of drowning, and don't know how to respond to drowning appropriately. Drowning is precisely defined as a type of respiratory impairment in which a liquid fills the lungs and makes it impossible to intake oxygen. Statistics show that on a worldwide level, drowning is the third most common cause of accidental death. The World Health Organization estimates that about 350,000 people die each year because of drowning.

It's important to note that drowning is entirely avoidable, and near-drowning is treatable. In fact, the top cause of drowning is simply not knowing how to swim. Not knowing how to swim and getting into the water is always a bad idea, but most claimed that there was no intention to get into the water. Boating and fishing often put people in a position where they are subject to falling into deep water and may not have life-saving protective equipment or the skill set to avoid drowning.

The absolute best thing you can do to avoid drowning altogether is to take swim classes. Even adults can benefit from swim classes, especially if they're going to be in situations with strong currents, rapids, deep water, or natural flowing waters. But don't worry, here we're going to cover exactly how to handle and near-drowning whether or not the injured person has experienced swimming.

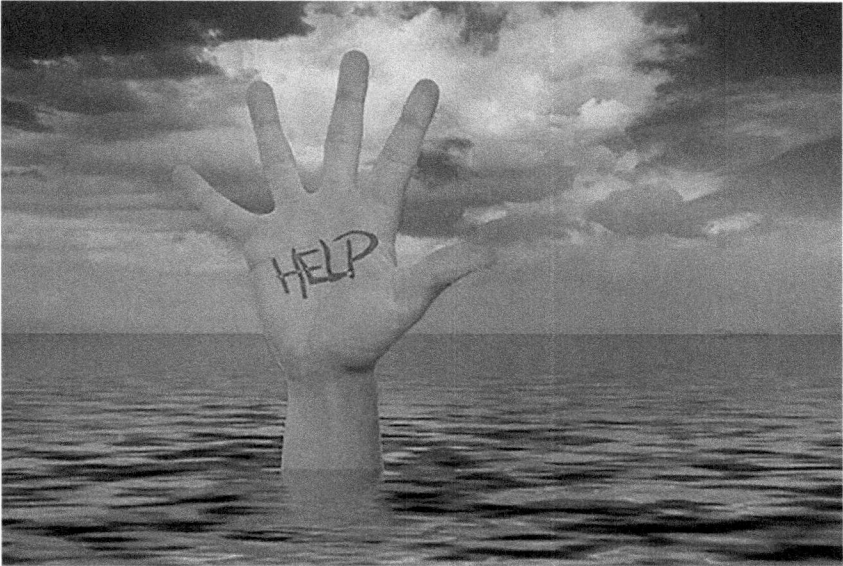

How to Identify if Someone is Drowning

The reason that drowning is the second most common unintentional injury that leads to the deaths of children between one and fourteen is that people don't know how to recognize the signs of drowning. Many initially believe that they would see someone in distress, kicking, maybe crying out for help, and someone clearly scared. That is not what drowning looks like.

Drowning is a silent death that takes between four and six minutes of the victim receiving no oxygen.

Drowning is almost always preventable if anyone is watching the water and realizes that someone is not coming up for air.

The most common sign of drowning is head-bobbing, the victim may be pushing their head above the water line just enough to gasp for air, but not enough to scream for help. Their arms and legs will be in the water. Another common sign is that the person drowning will have their head tilted far back to get more of their airway open to take in air.

Additionally, if you see someone with hair covering their eyes, it can be a good sign that they're drowning. While swimming, most people will naturally push their hair out of their face, but while in panic mode, that isn't a thought that crosses their mind. Additionally, if you can see a person's eyes, and it seems as though they're drowning, they may be looking into space, or their eyes may be glossed over.

If you ask a person that seems to be drowning if they are alright or okay and you don't get a response, then you need to take immediate action to get them out of the water.

How to Get Someone Out of the Water Safely

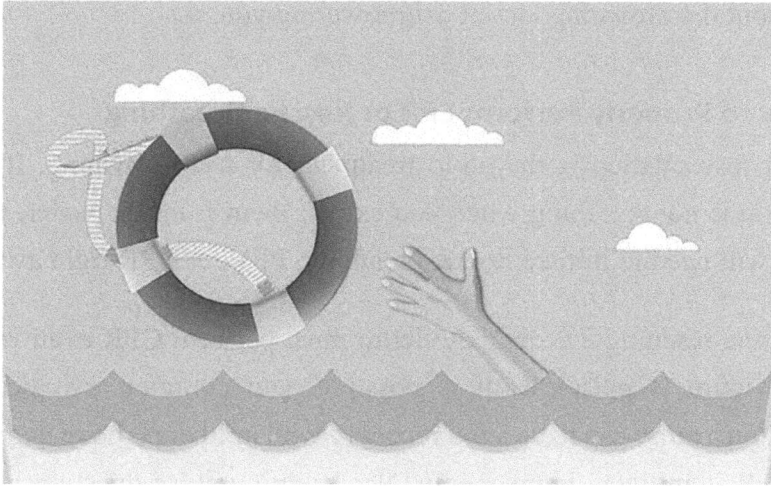

Many people have become secondary victims of drowning because they immediately jumped into the water. You may need to jump into the water, but your first approach needs to involve an object.

Get a sturdy object such as a branch, pole, flotation device, or similar object, and place it directly in front of the drowning person. The human body's instincts when drowning is to use the arms in a manner that looks similar to climbing a ladder. Placing a sturdy object in front of them will give them something to grab hold of, and you can reel them in.

If using an object to extract the person from the water does not work, then you may need to grab them from the water manually. While doing this, attempt to anchor yourself to something solid or unmoving as drowning victims often pull down the rescuer. Holding onto the boat, ladder, deck, or even another nearby person can give you enough weight to grab the person who is drowning and pull back without the drowning victim overpowering you.

How to Properly Perform CPR or Rescue Breathing

CPR resuscitation is the go-to treatment for near-drowning. If the person is not breathing when you extract them from the water, then you will need to initiate rescue breathing, PPV, or CPR right away.

Anyone rescuing a drowning victim must perform CPR even when the victim is pulseless. It is possible, and common that people without a pulse can have a full recovery with mild or no brain damage if CPR is initiated immediately. Not having a pulse does not mean the victim is beyond saving. You should continue these efforts for at least 30-minutes unless the person regains the ability to breathe on their own before that time.

Rescue breathing is what most people will do in response to drowning, especially if they're not trained in CPR. CPR is the preferred method when the person has no pulse. If a person has a pulse but is not breathing, perform rescue breathing by doing the following:

1. Place the person on their back, lying flat.

2. Put your palm on the person's forehead then, with your other hand, pull their chin away from their spine, opening their airway.

3. Check if the chest rises

4. Listen at their mouth for breathing

5. If there is no breath, then proceed.

6. Pinch the person's nose closed

7. Seal your mouth over their open mouth. If you have a faceguard or protective barrier, use it. If you can't open their mouth, breathe directly into their nose. For small children, you may need to breathe over their nose and mouth.

8. Give a deep breath into the victim's mouth for a one-second count. This is not the method for children under 1-year of age.

9. If their chest rose with the first breathe, repeat the one-second breathe again.

10. If their chest did not rise, tilt their head back, then tuck the chin down, and try again.

11. Repeat rescue breaths at ten breaths per minute, or one breath every six seconds, with chest compressions. Chest compressions should be almost constant, with 100-120 compressions happening per minute.

For Infants follow steps up until step seven, and then instead of step eight, follow:

• Two small or gentle puffs of air lasting for one second with at least two seconds of rest between puffs.

- If the chest rises, continue puffs.

- If the chest does not rise, tilt their head back, and chin down and try again.

- For infants, give two gentle breaths after a series of 30 chest compressions. Chest compressions must be fast.

How to Determine if this is an Emergency

Every instance of drowning is an emergency. If someone is crying out for help and making a splash in the water, then it's likely that they aren't drowning.

Dry Drowning and Secondary Drowning Symptoms

Dry drowning most commonly happens in children, but about 95% of children are perfectly fine after they fall in the water or even experience near-drowning. Less than 5% of children experience dry drowning. That doesn't mean that there should be any complacency in terms of watching for symptoms of dry drowning and taking immediate action to get help if dry drowning does happen.

Dry drowning and another term, secondary drowning, both result from trauma that happened during the drowning instant. Dry drowning can set in within an hour of inhaling water, and after that first hour, you're likely in the clear. Secondary drowning, however, can happen anywhere from the time of drowning to 48 hours afterward. The most dangerous window is within the first 24 hours of resuscitation.

Secondary drowning looks a lot more like real drowning because the lungs of the victim do fill with water. Both secondary drowning and dry drowning can be fatal.

Dry Drowning Symptoms and Response

Initially, the symptoms of dry drowning will include difficulty speaking or breathing, irritability, coughing, complaining of chest pain, and sleepiness. If the person is having trouble breathing, it's important to monitor them carefully. Try to keep the victim calm and to help them relax the muscles around their windpipe. The only treatment or response for dry drowning is to get them to immediate medical attention. They may need specialized equipment to keep their windpipe open, to clear liquid from their lungs, or to administer oxygen.

Secondary Drowning Symptoms and Response

Symptoms of secondary drowning include vomiting, coughing, difficulty breathing, fever, and even diarrhea. Treating a secondary drowning also requires specialized equipment. Often it requires a full ventilation system and a persistent feed of oxygen.

What to Do with Drowning

The most important thing to do when handling a drowning victim is to immediately begin rescue breathing with compressions, otherwise known as CPR. This is a life-saving tactic, and the American Health Association recommends CPR or rescues breathing with compression for all victims of drowning.

1. Extract the victim from the water immediately, using an object if possible.

2. Immediately begin rescue breathing.

3. When performing chest compressions, interlock your fingers with the heel of one hand over the back of the other hand.

4. When performing chest compressions, align your hands over the center of their chest.

5. When performing chest compressions, align your shoulders over your hands and keep your arms straight. Use your weight, and release pressure, but don't move your hands unless you're performing breaths.

6. Lift your fingers when performing compressions.

7. Continue rescue breathing for at least 30 minutes. Some victims have resumed breathing after 90 minutes of rescue breathing.

Using this method for rescue breathing and resuscitation can drastically change the outcome of the incident. If you can contact 911, then follow all of the instructions of the operator. If someone nearby is certified in CPR or Rescue Breathing, then allow them to take over. Never push yourself into a situation that deprives the patient of having a more qualified person working on them. Additionally, if you know that you're going to be spending long periods near water, then you should consider taking courses and becoming certified. One near-drowning experience is often enough to push people to get certified before their next excursion into the backcountry or wilderness. Even frequent beach campers should consider CPR or Red Cross training certifications.

You should also expect:

- Foaming at both the mouth and nose

- Vomiting

- Coughing or sputtering

- The victim fighting to sit up or roll over when they resume breathing

What Not to Do with Near Drowning

There are a few things that happen when handling a drowning victim that can make the situation worse. However, those things are far and few between. First, don't jump right into deep water in an attempt to save a drowning victim, especially if you are not a strong swimmer. The correct way of handling drowning or near-drowning is always to attempt to use an object to pull the victim up first. Then jump in if an object is unavailable or ineffective. Second, do not attempt to sit the victim up or pat them on the back as it may disrupt the water that's in their lungs and stomach in a more damaging way. Third, if you are approaching a drowning victim in the water, approach them from behind.

When it comes to giving treatment, don't assume that the lack of a pulse or that no signs of breathing mean the person is lost. Often people who initiate CPR without any signs of breathing or a pulse can revive and successfully resuscitate the injured person.

Finally, don't assume that once the person is breathing, the danger is gone. Dry drowning, secondary drowning, lung infections, and complications from oxygen loss are all possible issues you may face in the upcoming hours. Typically, you can declare the patient as "safe" 48 hours after the rescue.

Aftercare

Aftercare for drowning almost always requires medical attention. Even just getting to a nearby ranger station can be critical because if dry drowning or secondary drowning does ensue, there's nothing you can do in the wilderness. If you can get to a ranger station, or even better an Urgent Care Center, they will likely monitor the person for six to 24 hours after the drowning incident. That is the window of time in which dry drowning would happen, and after that time, the recovering patient would likely be released.

The other reason that taking medical attention is important after a drowning incident is that the quality of water may lead to infection in the lungs. Poor quality water can often lead to bacteria getting into the lungs, and bacteria can manifest into an infection.

Finally, there is the chance of a blood clot getting into the lungs and causing further health complications. This is called pulmonary edema and often happens to middle-aged people, but it's also a complication of drowning. It happens because of the body's response during the drowning process, and pulmonary edema can happen in a later four to the six-hour window after drowning.

The risks of dry drowning, infection, and blood clots or pulmonary edema are very low. However, no one should take the chance that these rare occurrences wouldn't happen to them. Most people believe that they won't experience drowning, so the belief that you wouldn't experience infection, dry drowning, or blood clots should be thrown out the window. While it can certainly be a pain to get to a medical facility when you're in the wilderness or the backwoods, it doesn't mean that you shouldn't try. If you are more than 24-hours away from a medical center or a ranger station, then you should still take the movement to evacuate.

The patient may be seemingly making a full recovery and just a little shaken up from experience, but if someone nearly drowned on your excursion, it's time to pack up and head back towards civilization. If they do show signs of any of these complications, you may be within range for emergency medical transport to reach you before those complications progress and become life-threatening.

Chapter 5

Burns

On a very general level, burns are terrifying. But, of the most common injuries, burns are not only easily avoidable but often easily treatable. In fact, the American Burn Organization declares the survival rate for burn victims is 96.8%, with the highest risk of non-survival being from residential fires. Perhaps the first most important thing to do is not to panic. If the person is still exposed to flame, put the flame out immediately. Stop drop and roll method is best. If the person caught in the fire cannot or does not calm down, then take a jacket, blanket, sleeping bag, or blanket, get them to the ground and smother the fire.

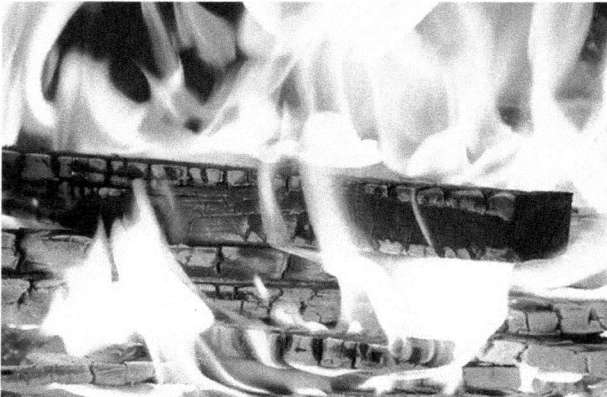

Most Common Camping Injury

Roofers are the second leading cause of injury at campsites, often because of the open fires, cooking with unfamiliar equipment, and using fires or stoves placed on the ground. These are all preventable with proper planning and awareness of your surroundings. Unfortunately, camping often comes with roughhousing, alcohol, and any variety of other substances or behaviors that have people more relaxed than usual.

Burns can happen from handling hot pots, boiling water, fire, and even primitive tools that may get unexpectedly hot. Burns most frequently happen on hands and feet, and extremity burns are often the easiest to treat but may require more monitoring.

Now, most first aid kits will have a burn dressing, and the appropriate gel or treatment for burns, but we have some go-to options for how to handle these extremely common injuries without all the proper resources as well.

Assess the Damage: How Much Surface Area and What Degree

The burn damage that you see initially is not the full extent of the damage. Burns will continue to worsen if they are not treated immediately. The heat retained in the tissue can cause further damage hours or even days after the skin was exposed to fire or extreme heat.

But, if you know the general degree of the burn, and the surface area, you can take greater steps to provide full first aid to the burn and reduce the likelihood of extended injury. Rachel elements not only help direct people to treat them properly but can help people understand how to monitor the injury, and when it's time to evacuate.

How to Tell How Much Surface Area of the Skin was Damaged

If a burn damages more than 10% of the total surface area of the skin, then it's likely the person will need professional medical treatment within the near future. When you're handling this much surface area, there's the likelihood that the person will go into shock, and they are more likely to sustain infection. But how can you tell how much surface area was damaged?

The rule of palms says that the size of your palm is roughly 1% of your body's total surface skin area. To estimate the percentage of a surface area burned, count how many times your palm can cover the burned skin.

The rule of palms is not the definitive answer, but it is a great way to get an estimate on how much burn area you're working with.

Placement

Placement of the burn is perhaps more important than the percentage of surface area covered. Although burnt palms and forearms are among the most common, they're also the most troublesome. The second most common placement for a burn is feet, and that is also quite troublesome.

If you're dealing with a burn on either the person's hands or feet, then you should make sure that you carefully watch the injury and evacuate at any sign of infection.

If you are dealing with a burn on the Torso or trunk region, you'll need to monitor the injury, but generally, you will end up checking the injury less frequently than hand and foot burns.

Burns to the face is immediately severe and does call for evacuation because the patient may have inhaled a high amount of heat, and it may have done damage to the esophagus and lungs.

If you noticed that the burn injury goes all the way around a limb, for example, completely encasing a forearm, you should also consider evacuation if the burn is of the second or third-degree.

How to Determine the Burn Degree

Understanding burn degrees is a bit more complex than most people give credit to. First, there are two sets of vocabulary that apply to the same burn evaluation process. First-degree burns are also called outer layer burns and are typically mild. They are painful, they can result in reddening of the area, and it may be visible that the skin came into contact with a very hot item.

Second-degree burns are also called partial thickness Burns. This means that the top of the skin and the layer of skin underneath were affected by the burn. Second-degree burns are often identified by blistering. Second-degree burns are among the most common, because people often experience these when cooking at home, or even in most workplaces.

Third-degree burns is called full-thickness Burns, and they affect not only both layers of the skin but also the tissue underneath. You can identify a third-degree burn by recognizing blackness or charring of the skin, or even the remaining skin may be chalky white. Often third-degree burns may be painful in the beginning and then quickly drop in pain level. If the person does not report any pain, it may be typical of a third-degree burn. The most serious degrees of burns are often reported as painless.

In both the second and third-degree burns you'll likely see the skin peeling back, the person may go into shock, there will likely be immediate swelling in the injured area, and the person will likely experience pain.

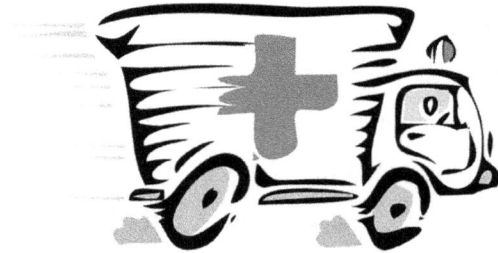

Treating Shock

The symptoms of shock include the person going clammy, having a cold sweat, experiencing weakness, going pale, having bluish or purple lips, experiencing blue-tinged fingernails, and a noted drop in alertness.

Shock during a burn can happen for one of two reasons, the severity of the burn can cause someone to go into shock, and this is only common with third-degree or deep tissue burns. The second reason that someone would go into shock during the burn is because of blood loss, which also indicates that the burn is very severe and requires immediate first aid attention.

Now you can proactively help to prevent a burnt person from going into shock. Take these steps to help prevent shock if you're noticing the early symptoms such as disorientation, confusion, thirst, rapid breathing, dizziness, blue-tinged lips are fingernails, nervousness, or agitation.

To treat and prevent the onset shock:

1. If conscious, lay the injured person flare and elevate the legs six to eight inches.

   a. If the person is unconscious, then turn them on their side with their head turned to that same direction.

2. Remove wet clothing.

3. Give small doses of lightly sugared water. Warm or air-temperature water is preferable.

4. Keep the injured person in a shaded area.

5. Maintain their body heat, even in midday; they may need a blanket, shock can cause the body to cool rapidly.

When a person is in shock, they may vomit or bleed from the mouth and may need resuscitation. If someone is bleeding from the mouth or vomiting, then roll them onto their side, unless it's suspected that they have a spinal or neck injury. Refer to chapter 4, or the end of this book, for full information on how to perform a CPR.

How to Determine if this is an Emergency

Often the only time that you'll need to consider evacuation is if the person experienced third-degree burns, needs medical help for pain management, or when second or third-degree burns covering more than 10% of their total body surface area. Even in the backwoods, this is fairly uncommon. For short of falling straight into the fire pit, most people have likely sustained burns from nearby hot or extremely cold objects.

Now it appears that there are symptoms of any airway burns, including coughing, rattling breath, respiratory disease visibly singed facial hairs. It would be best to consider evacuation to get prompt medical attention or get closer to medical professionals.

Perhaps the bigger initial concern for most is the opportunity of infection. If you've burned your hands, feet, face, or groin, then you might consider evacuation simply to get proper wound care. In most situations like these, there is not much that medical professionals can do other than dress the wound and manage the pain.

What to Do with Burn Wounds

Typically burn treatment is very straightforward. Follow these steps:

1. Remove the clothing and all jewelry or restrictive items near the burn. For example, if you are burned on your forearm, you would still need to remove rings, as the entire limb will likely swell to some degree.

2. Reduce the heat with cool, but not cold, water. Do not immerse the burn in water.

Placing a cold object on a burn can severely damage the tissue and skin area even more than the burn itself. Use clean, preferably potable water that is just below room temperature and is not "ice-cold" or chilled to cool the burn. If running natural water is your only option, then use it; otherwise, attempt to use bottled or filtered water.

3. Clean the burn.

Cleaning a burn can be a daunting task, but the best approach is with simple, gentle antibacterial soap. Standard, unscented, hand soap is best, but scented soap or antibacterial hand wipes in your first aid kit can work as well. Be gentle when washing over open areas of skin, and don't 'scrub' or aggressively pull at charred skin areas.

4. Moisturize and Cover

First, note that first and second-degree burns may not require any covering. You should not 'pop' blisters, but if a blister has opened on a second-degree burn, then be sure to cover it. Second, keep in mind that burned skin and tissue will attempt to adhere to nearly all forms of cloth. You must moisturize the wounded area with Neosporin, antibacterial or antibiotic gel, or even petroleum jelly such as Aquaphor or Vaseline.

Below is a list of commonly accepted 'home' remedies for moisturizing burn wounds. If you do not have Neosporin or similar, refer to that list.

This will prevent the skin from sticking to the bandage. Finally, the bandage should be non-stick, use gauze before you use Band-Aids.

If you don't have clean gauze, then a clean tee-shirt or fabric is the next best option. It is better to cover burn wounds with an alternative fabric than it would be to leave them open.

5. Treat the Pain

The pain is often the last thing to address when handling burns. The person may feel more or less pain than surrounding people would expect, and extreme burns often come without any pain at all. It's best to use over-the-counter pain relievers, including Acetaminophen or Ibuprofen, to reduce swelling and relieve pain.

Recommended "Home" Remedies for Those with Limited Resources

It doesn't matter if you were burned by an open flame or handling a cast iron pan while presiding over a campfire. Burns have happened since before people were around, and we've largely found what works and what doesn't work in regard to Natural or home remedies. While some home remedies, such as butter, have been proven to do more damage than good, these are the options that can help soothe the pain, calm the damaged tissue, and help the wound begin to heal.

Use these home remedies if items such as Neosporin or antibacterial gel or not available use aloe vera or honey.

What Not to Do with Burn Wounds

Many common mistakes happened with burn wounds, but all of these are entirely avoidable. Unfortunately, the reason that so many of these mistakes are common is that they seem like the right approach, or they seem like common sense. In fact, many of these were recommended practice until the last few years or the last few decades. For example, only a few decades ago, people would often recommend popping blisters, now we know that that can open the wound to infection.

Here is a complete list of what not to do with a burn wound.

Do NOT:

- Put butter on a burn wound. Or any other oily-substance.

- Ice the burn

- Only use enough water to clean the wound. Instead, make sure that you run water over the wound to cool the underlayers of skin or tissue.

- Expose the wound to open air or sun. In other words, don't let the wound "air out."

- Pop blisters.

- Remove clothing or cloth stuck to an open burn wound.

- Put toothpaste on the wound.

Aftercare

If the burn was a second or first-degree and showed no evidence of charring or turning white, then you can likely care for it completely at home. For third-degree burns, make sure to schedule a follow-up appointment with a primary care physician.

To treat first and second-degree burns on your own, you'll want to follow these steps:

1. Use running water to soak-off bandages. Do not attempt to remove a dry bandage.

2. Wash the wound three or four times per day with mild soap and cool running water.

3. Follow each washing with cream or moisturizing substance, preferably an antibacterial one or a topical antibiotic.

4. Gently massage the area during healing. In a week or so, the burn is completely healed.

Keep in mind always that burns can easily become infected. Always be on the lookout for the development of pus pockets, changes in color, and changes in smell. Check and wash the wound often, the skin will heal in its own time.

If you experience burns over frequently used muscle areas, then you might ask your general practitioner about physical therapy. Even if you have no problem treating the burn injury on your own, and healing in the week or so after the injury, you might still need physical therapy. Many people struggle to continue to flex and use the tissue that was damaged during the burn. Get on that the most common areas for burns are the hands. You'll likely need some form of physical therapy, especially if you didn't take time to gently massage the area and continue using the hand as normal during the healing process. After a burn, the muscles and skin can heal any more restrictive or tightened state then what is natural for that muscle or skin tissue. Often physical therapy that addresses hand burns will include carefully flexing individual fingers and working the hand muscles both individually and together to regain control and movement.

First and second-degree burns are often something you can handle entirely on your own. Unless you see clear color changes in your skin from the burn, signs of infection, or signs of charring along their flesh, your aftercare may be as simple as keeping the wound clean, moist, and covered. In any case, if you haven't any concern for how your burn wound is healing, then arrange for an appointment with a general practitioner or family practitioner. Burns are so common that you probably don't need a specialist unless your doctor recommends physical therapy.

Chapter 6

Broken and Dislocated Bones

How familiar are you with human anatomy? Can you name the bones in various parts of the body? Are you aware of which sections in the human body have two bones and which have one or structural support? The most common answers to these questions are "no." most people cannot name intricate bones in the body, most are not familiar with different types of fractures, and most are not aware of what areas have two bones and which have singular bones. So, if at this very moment, you are worried or even panicking that you don't have the knowledge to address a broken bone in this emergency situation, take a breath. With very basic knowledge, you can treat a fracture or a dislocation in the wild.

Broken bones and dislocated joints can come with a more than fair amount of pain. Not only are these injuries painful, but they often can incapacitate the injured person. These injuries are traumatic not only on the injured person but also on the entire wilderness group.

How to Tell if the Bone is Broken or Dislocated

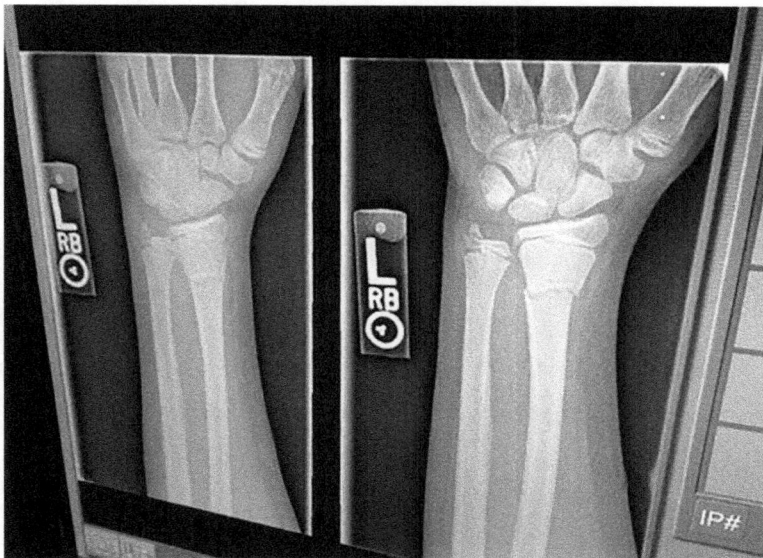

A common question, and a well-justified one, is, "How do you know if the phone is broken?" Most people can go their entire lives without encountering a broken bone or having to treat one. Unfortunately, the most common signs of broken bones are often signs of sprains, strains, and general soft tissue damage. Clearly, a broken bone is far more serious than a sprain, so a lot of the information you need to detect if a bone is broken will come from the injured person directly.

First, Look for the three common signs of a broken bone. Fractures, or broken bones, will often, with quickly onset pain, swelling, and deformity around the limb. You may notice bulges or sections around the bone that just doesn't seem right. These are also the common signs of a sprain, so move on to evaluating other possible signs of a broken bone. Other symptoms can include bruising around the area, which is also common with a sprained, and tenderness to the touch, also present with sprained injuries.

What may be the ultimate answer to deciding if a bone is broken or not, is talking directly to the injured person. Do they feel a grinding near the injury? Did they feel or hear a snap or grind as the injury happened? Are they able to flex or move hands or feet that are past the point of injury?

Other common signs that a bone is broken and that the injury is not simply a sprain, is that the injured person may feel sick, faint, dizzy, or maybe even go into shock as a result of the pain from the injury. However, some people may not report any pain and may feel as though they just stretch the muscle too far.

Then, there are other times when it is very evident that a bone is broken. For example, if the bone is protruding from the skin, there isn't any question about whether the bone is broken or not.

Determining if a joint is dislocated is much easier than attempting to determine if the phone is broken. In the event of dislocation, the joint will simply not be in a normal position. The person may not have any range of motion or movement with the joint, or any control over anything's possible joint.

Unlike broken bones, dislocations are always painful. The person may not be able to put any weight on it or stand someone touching the joint. Additionally, injured persons May report a numbness or tingling sensation as a joint or past the affected joint.

How to Determine if this is an Emergency

You may have noticed that broken bones are really pushed to the bottom of the list in terms of emergency room priority. Most medical professionals don't consider them an emergency unless the phone is projecting from the skin, or if any area below the injury is cold, blue, clammy, or pale.

If there is severe bleeding, then this is an emergency, and you need to evacuate immediately. Additionally, if there are signs of infection, such as redness or warmth around the injury site then evacuate as soon as possible.

Most bones will also require a medical professional or to properly cast or set the brake. However, you can likely establish a high-quality splint in the wilderness and essentially take your time to get into a medical office. You may even be able to call and set up an appointment with your primary care physician for one of the upcoming days. Usually, you do not have to go to an emergency room for a cast.

Most dislocations will require a medical professional, although some people are comfortable attempting to reconnect the joint themselves. If you don't feel comfortable attempting to re-establish a connection for dislocation, then evacuate and seek medical attention. When it comes to re-establishing a connection and a dislocation injury, hesitancy can often lead to further damage.

What to Do with Broken Bones

Handling fractures is one thing that most people feel they can't do, but the process is very straightforward and easy to manage. If the force of the injury fractured the bone, then you'll need to find a way to reduce the weight placed on the body part, reduce the pain, and reduce the swelling. At this time, you're not worrying about setting the bone properly or establishing it to heal on its own. In fact, if you do this, then a medical professional may have to later re-break the bone to set it properly. The only thing you're trying to do at this point is to properly splint the injury so that it is manageable and not prone to infection or further damage.

The traditional methods of treating fractures include splinting the injury in the position that it's currently in. If you are in the backcountry or the general wilderness, then it's likely that you are probably hours or days away from a medical facility. With that time frame in mind, the traditional methods of treating a fracture aren't useful in the wilderness. You will need to carefully manipulate the fracture to get it into a normal position to protect the structure of the muscles, tissue, nerves, and circulatory system.

To give a bit more insight, if you broke your leg at home you would splint it in the position that you broke it in and go to an urgent care center or arrange for a doctor's appointment. In the backcountry, if you do this is a muscle, nerves, and blood flow will all suffer for an extended period of time.

Follow these steps to treat a fracture in the wilderness:

1. Gently grasp the limb closer to the center of the body or nearest joint. For example, a broken shin would call for grasping the bottom of the knee, but a broken thigh bone would call for grasping the upper thigh close to the trunk of the body.

2. Apply steady traction or pressure to the part of the fracture that is furthest away from the area where it should attach. To do this, use your free hand.

3. Use only slow, downward, and gentle pressure. Do not attempt to pull up or to the side. Have the injured person angle themselves so that all pressure is applied downward.

4. Once the limb is back in its correct position, the injured person should have some relief. If the person complains of more pain, then the movement was not done properly.

5. Hold the limb in its correct position; do not let go.

6. Evaluate the blood flow, sensation, and movement below the injury. The person may not be able to wiggle toes or move fingers, but they should feel sensation and should have normal blood flow to the area.

7. Apply splint.

Applying a Splint

If a bone was protruding, or if the person experienced an open fracture, then you'll need to clean the wound gently before you apply the splint. Usually, these are for long bone fractures, and you may have seen more damage done to the skin by pushing the bone back into the body. That is normal for these types of injuries, but, cleaning the wound and keeping it covered can be critical to prevent infection.

Keep in mind before applying a splint that it should be snug, but it should not restrict the circulation or cause any pain. If the injured person complains that the splint is too tight, loosen it. Additionally, quality splints will have two or more straps around the fracture. They should also use padding to prevent discomfort and remain effective.

Different splint shapes:

- Long backboard - meant for long-bone injuries such as thigh and upper arm breaks.

- Short backboard - meant for bones broken near a joint, or for dislocated joints.

- Air splint - circular-shaped splint that should wrap entirely around the limb.

- Half ring splint - circular-shaped splint that cradles the underside of a short bone break.

- Gutter splints - similar to the half ring splint but cradles from the extended ring and pinky fingers down past the wrist or even to the elbow.

- Different Types of Splints include:

- Rigid splints - improvised splints made from wood, cardboard, and wire. Usually in the shape of an air splint, backboard, board splint, or a cardboard splint.

- Soft splints - made from rolled blankets, towels, and other soft materials. Often using yarn, twine, or wire to keep the splint secure.

- Improvised slings - used for extremities made from clothes, pack straps, branches, and more.

- Stirrup splints - Used for the ankle and shin, calls for wrapping padding under the heel and securing it in a stirrup shape. Secure the sides of the ankle and immobilize the joint.

- Double sugar tong splint - essential two stirrup splints applied first across the back of the elbow toward the wrist, and then from the bottom of the elbow toward the shoulder. This splint should immobilize the wrist and elbow.

Keep in mind that the point of splinting is to immobilize the area completely. Aim to immobilize the joint above and below the injury, if possible. It may seem impossible to immobilize a hip, but shoulders are easily immobilized or greatly inconvenienced at least.

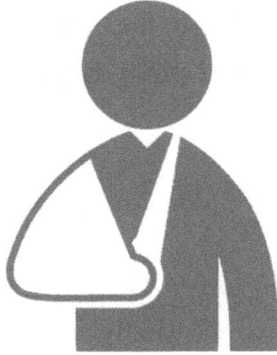

- If the *upper arm* is broken, use a splint to secure the bone into its natural position. Then, use a sling to pull the entire arm close to the body, angling the elbow at 90-degrees if uninjured, and, if possible, immobilize the wrist as well to reduce the inclination to reach and flex the wrist.

- If the *forearm* is broken, immobilize the elbow with a double sugar tong splint, and the wrist with a gutter splint shape.

- If the *thigh bone* is broken, then splint it with a rigid splint with a long backboard to immobilize the entire leg.

- If either *shin bone* is broken, then use a circular or half-ring splint and immobilize both the knee and the ankle.

- If *joints* are broken, then immobilize them in a circular splint, and immobilize the entire limb. For example, with a knee, you would place a circular splint on the knee then use a longboard splint to immobilize the entire leg.

As you make the splint, remember to splint both above and below where you believe the fracture site is, and to pad the splints thoroughly to reduce any discomfort.

What to Do with Dislocations

Dislocations can be extremely painful as they are the separation of bone joints, which can lead to bones going out of their alignment, and complete loss of use of the limb after the dislocation. Setting the bones back into proper alignment is the only course of treatment for dislocation, and the process of setting is sometimes called reduction. You want to use a variety of methods that involves your weight and pulling the bones back together safely.

Putting the bones back into their proper place should ease the pain and allow the limb to function normally again. The joint should resume normal function immediately, although some of the pain may stick around for a while.

- For *shoulder dislocation*: don't try to push the joint back into place. Splint the shoulder by bringing the elbow against the ribs in a sling and make the patient as comfortable as possible. There are far too many nerves and the high possibility of other damage to attempt to reconnect a shoulder in the wilderness.

- For *dislocated knee/kneecaps*: easy to identify as kneecap will visibly be on the outside of the knee. Apply pressure to straighten out the leg completely while guiding the kneecap back into place with your thumb or palm of your hand. Then, apply a cold treatment, and splint to immobilize the leg.

- For a *dislocated elbow*: this can be extremely painful for the patient, and restoring an elbow often requires two people. When you only have one person, have them lie flat, on their stomach, a car or table, and gently and slowly pull the wrist down while guiding the elbow with your thumb back into place. With two people, it is similar, but then you have two hands to guide the elbow back into place, which has a much higher success rate.

- For a *dislocated knee*: the process is generally faster than other methods of reduction but should still be done fairly slowly. Have on person hold the shin stable, and the second person should carefully pull the ankle down, away from the shin, and then twist and guide it back into place.

What Not to Do with Broken or Dislocated Bones

There are a few particular things that you should avoid doing when handling a broken or dislocated. First, if at all possible, don't move the injured person. Additionally, if it's the leg that's broken, try to keep them in one position. In fact, if the leg is broken, then you should explore options to have Emergency Medical Services come to you. You can cause a lot of damage by transporting someone with a broken leg, and it's not always clear if there's an extensive injury done to the tissue, circulatory system, or muscles in the area. If you know that you can get to Ranger Station, then get help and bring medical assistance to the injured person. If you're truly in the backwoods or out in the country and have no hope of getting medical help to you, then craft a lift or a drag. The idea is to pull the injured person rather than expecting them to coordinate any movement.

Even when the injury seems really urgent, don't rush the injured person to move faster than they're physically capable of handling. Even people with broken arms a likely need to move at a much slower pace, and although medical attention could seem extremely urgent, moving at a comfortable pace is more important unless there is clear traumatic injury.

Aftercare

After reducing a dislocated joint, or splinting a broken bone, you still want to have a medical professional look at the injury and likely cast it. Casting is not something that should be done by anyone without specialized training. However, your splint could have drastically changed the injured person's pain level and their recovery.

Aftercare will often involve physical therapy, after weeks of not using the limb at all. They may have a limited range of motion forever, and there's likely nothing you could have done in the wilderness to have helped them prepare for a complete recovery. Additionally, aftercare may involve surgery. If, during the reduction of a dislocated joint, when there was any damage to the muscle or nerves, then a medical professional may need to perform surgery to correct the damage. Just the same, if there was damage done while you were correcting or splinting a broken phone, or if you did not set the phone correctly, a medical professional might need to re-break the bone, reset it, and begin the healing process all over again.

Chapter 7

Head Injuries

Head trauma frequently happens in the wild and for a wide variety of reasons. From falls to stumbling into unforeseen objects or obstacles, you should definitely know how to treat a head wound when the time calls for it. There is the chance that any head wound could be very serious and even lead to death. The short and long term damage may be something that depends on the immediate response and care for the wounded.

What is troublesome is that it's common for people to confuse the signs of head trauma with the signs of other common wilderness illnesses such as altitude sickness. There are a few primary types of head wounds you can expect to encounter in the wilderness or backcountry, and it can be critical to take immediate and decisive action. Some treatments won't result in the immediate need for evacuation. It all depends on the severity of the injury and what resources you have available to treat the injured person.

Recent research shows that head injuries are the third most common location for injuries sustained in the wilderness. The most common cause of these types of injuries includes falling, which is responsible for about half of the head injuries and being struck by an object.

From Concussions to Coup-Contrecoup

These injuries can happen become of a fall or even just getting knocked on the head with someone else's equipment. If it looks like it's just a goose-egg, then you might be fine, but it's always best to carefully evaluate the injury and the patient. It's important to remember that often head and brain injuries don't show any external symptoms. Sometimes symptoms are so difficult to detect that the person only learns about the damage associated with the trauma weeks or months later.

Read through these common head injuries that happen in the wilderness, then we'll get into how to determine if it's a serious head injury.

Concussions

Know the signs of a concussion, but also keep in mind that a concussion can be rather mild to very serious. Many people experience concussions and have no idea that they experienced concussions at all. In the wild, it's always important to clearly rule out the possibility of a concussion or to treat the concussion appropriately.

The symptoms of a concussion include:

- Headache

- Nausea
- Difficulty balancing
- Dizziness
- Fatigue
- Sensitivity to light or sound
- A "buzzing" or tingling sensation
- Mental fog
- Feeling as if they're moving slow
- Trouble concentration
- Forgetfulness
- Confusions
- Taking a long time to answer questions
- Irritability
- Emotionally sad or over-expressive
- Overly sensitive
- Nervousness or anxiety

With a *mild concussion*, the person may be fully capable of walking, have no loss of consciousness, and may only present symptoms hours after the event. Most people with a mild concussion will need weeks or months to recover with additional mental and physical rest but often don't run the risk of developing further complications.

A *moderate concussion* will involve a temporary loss of consciousness, no memory of the traumatic event, and they may not remember the moments leading up to the event either. The injured person may still be able to walk, but without rest, the injury will probably progress to a severe concussion. Moderate concussions may come with visual symptoms such as a blood pooling beneath the scalp causing a "bubble" or cerebral spinal fluid (CSF) a clear or light yellow liquid, possibly tinged with blood, pooling in the ears.

A *severe concussion* may take 24 hours or more to present all the symptoms that would lead someone to believe that the injury is this serious. However, a person with a severe concussion will likely have clear visual damage or trauma such as a depressed skull fracture where the bone of the skull is caved inward, penetrating trauma, or clear CSF leaking from their ears and possibly their nose.

Both moderate and severe concussions can lead to intracranial pressure or ICP. It's a dangerous condition that requires immediate medical intervention. Typically, ICP after head trauma will come with seizures, and the person may move into a "funeral" type position where they lay flat with their wrists crossed over their chest. That position is often followed by throwing the hands down at the sides forcefully. This position is called 'Decerebrate posturing.' Decerebrate posturing is often followed by a change in breathing rate, as well as respiratory and cardiac arrest.

Coup-Contrecoup

Coup-contrecoup is occasionally present in hikers who may have fallen in one direction, and then injured the other side of their head as well. What happens in coup-contrecoup injuries is that the brain impacts one side of the interior of the skull, while additional damage is done to the other side of the skull. The brain may "rattle" between the two sides, and this injury might be serious. The brain will have contusions.

Usually, these injuries are not reversible but may require immediate medical intervention. The brain may be bleeding or swelling. Allow the patient to get some rest and plan for an evacuation. These injuries will almost always be easy to assess their severity. However, most medical professionals assess a coup-contrecoup injury that does not come with additional injuries such as fractures as mild traumatic brain injuries. You can detect a coup-contrecoup injury by witnessing a loss of consciousness and loss of memory after an injury that would have clearly rattled the brain.

Fractures

Skull fractures are very straightforward and often easy to detect. Unfortunately, they come with more severe symptoms and often demand immediate evacuation. Skull fracture will often have an obvious deformity such as a scalp wound, and depression, blood pooling beneath the scalp resulting in a bubble, and possible cerebral spinal fluid coming from the ears or nose. You must take care when attempting to assess a skull fracture as you don't want to present pressure over the fracture accidentally.

Skull fractures can often come with extreme brain damage, can come with ICP, which is life-threatening within 24 hours, may require surgery, and with some complications may lead to meningitis, which can also be life-threatening. Skull fractures are very serious, however, not every skull fracture will result in a loss of not every skull fracture will result in CSF fluid leaking, and not every skull fracture requires surgery.

Use the AVPU Scale

The AVPU scale serves to help people assess the person's level of brain function and alertness. It is often used as the indicator to determine when to evacuate, and how urgently the person or group needs to evacuate.

A indicates that the patient is awake. They may be awake and confused, but they are awake. It means that they don't need verbal or physical stimulus to have a conversation or engage in regular brain function.

V indicates that the person requires a verbal stimulus to interact and that their brain function may be slowing. This is equivalent to talking to a drunk person on the verge of passing out or a person that has mentally checked out. If you have to shout, "Hey, are you okay?" and they raise their eyes and issue some type of response, then they're at the "V" stage.

P indicates that the verbal stimulus didn't work, and the person requires pain stimulus to respond. Pain stimulus can be initiated by pinching the soft skin on the underside of the upper arm, or by roughly running your knuckles over their sternum. The response may be slight movement, verbal muttering, grunting, or even pushing your hand away.

U shows that the person is unresponsive. They may be a "u" and still show vital signs, but if the person is outright unresponsive to pain or verbal stimulus, then proceed with evacuating immediately. Always check for other injuries before moving the injured person, but at the "u" end of the scale, ICP can set in within a few hours, and the person may be in a life-threatening position before you can reach medical help.

Keep in mind that the person's level on the scale may change. Monitor the injured person every 2-4 hours and reconduct the scale to determine if their condition is improving or getting worse.

Remember that at any point that someone is unresponsive, you should take immediate evacuation measures.

An Alternative: The Glasgow Coma Scale

The Glasgow coma scale uses a number system to determine how serious a head injury is or is not. The scale follows this point system:

- 4 points for open eyes with blinking.

- 3 points for responding to speech or verbal stimulus.

- 2 points for responding to pain only

- 1 point for no response to visual, pain, or verbal stimulus

- 5 points for being well-oriented with speech

- 4 points for being confused but able to answer questions

- 3 points for responding but providing responses that don't make sense

- 2 points for speech that makes no sense or is incomprehensible

- 1 point for no response.

- 6 points for obeying commands to move (ex: lift your hand, touch your nose)

- 5 points for movement response to pain (brushing away a hand)

- 4 points for withdrawal to pain response

- 3 points for early posturing or flexing because of pain

- 2 points for decerebrate posturing (life-threatening)

- 1 point for no motor response

The totals should tell you how serious the head injury is and help you determine how to respond. If there is a score of 8 or lower, than the head injury is severe. If the score is between 9 and 12, then the head injury is moderate but needs medical attention. A score between 13 and 15 is a mild head injury, and there's likely no need to evacuate at that point.

These scores or scales are helpful, but they're not the only way to determine if the situation is an emergency. There are always additional factors to consider.

How to Determine if this is an Emergency

Diagnosing a brain or head trauma can be fairly straightforward, but you'll need to use your best judgment. First, always refer to the AVPU scale and use that as your primary guide to determine the seriousness of a head injury.

Now, if the trauma seems to be just a bump on the head, then it might not be an emergency. The biggest signs of an emergency are a "U" on the AVPU scale, or the presence of other injuries if those injuries are also severe. Sometimes the signs that a brain injury or head trauma is becoming worse is that the injured person may become aggressive or combative. If that behavior is out of character for them, then attempt to calm them, but do not restrain the person. Even medical professionals are slowing down on how often they use restraints when treating someone with head trauma. The sign of agitation or aggression is a huge red flag of a severe traumatic brain injury. The situation at this point is an emergency, and the injured person may not be aware that they're putting others at risk too.

The Presence of Other Injuries

Head trauma will often come along with simple cuts and bruising. That's fine and treatable with flesh wound treatment and ice. But there are often situations, especially while falling when hiking, that the head trauma could come hand in hand with a spinal injury, neck injury, and severe cuts.

Before performing any treatment, carefully survey the scalp and general head area for open wounds. Feel through thick or long hair for wetness. Additionally, use your fingertips to feel down the neck and spine gently. If anything feels out of place, do not move the victim, contact help, and, if necessary, engage a search and rescue team. If you are too far into the wilderness to leave and get help, then initiate emergency procedures to grab attention from possible search and rescue teams such as flares or smoke signals.

What to Do with Head Injuries

When it comes to treating head injuries, there are a lot of good general practices, but many others relate directly to specific situations. Here we will list out the general best practices first and then address specific situations or challenges.

Treating all head injuries:

- Evaluate the person's heart rate by counting the person's heart beats for 15 seconds and then multiplying that by 4 to determine the beats per minute.

  o A "normal" resting heart rate is often between 60-100 beats per minute, but athletes, the very young, and the elderly may go outside of that range.

  o Even the body position can change a heart rate.

  o You want to continue to monitor the heart rate periodically to watch for changes.

- Engage the person in conversation and ask questions to determine their level of confusion or disorientation. Do this often to gauge improvement as normal brain function can return quickly.

- Check on the injured person often, at least every 2-4 hours.

Concussion treatment:

- Minimize physical or mental exertion, allow the patient to rest and sleep.

- Wake the injured person every 2-4 hours to test alertness.

- Provide acetaminophen to reduce headache pain.

- Monitor for changes in symptoms and increase the evacuation rate if necessary.

- If there is persistent vomiting, help the victim sleep or rest, and begin evacuating immediately. Reduce physical or mental stress to the injured person during an evacuation.

- If there are any signs of ICP, do not wait to evacuate, evacuate immediately the situation is life-threatening.

What to do in one-off situations:

- If the person is in a dangerous area, then move them. Spine damage happens in a small percentage of people with head trauma, and it may be more important to get them out of danger than to stabilize the spine. Additionally, newer first-aid practices call for spine protection or careful handling rather than outright stabilization when the victim must be moved.

- If there are signs of shock, then treat for shock by getting the victim onto their back and elevating their feet. If the injured person is not responsive, then roll them onto their side and do not elevate their feet.

- If the person has a cut or gash, then clean the wound gently and bandage it as you would handle a flesh wound, see chapter 2.

- If the person comes in at a "P" or a "U" on the scale, then evacuate from the wilderness immediately.

What Not to Do with Head Injuries

Most of what we know now about what not to do with head injuries are associated with "old wives tales" and home remedies that were probably based on medical advice from many years ago. Here is a complete list of what not to do in the event of a head injury.

Do NOT:

- Keep a person with a head injury awake for fear of concussion. The brain needs rest to repair itself. It is okay for people with head injuries to nap or outright sleep as long as someone checks in on them and wakes them up every hour to gauge their alertness.

- Force a person to sit up after a head injury, allow them to lie down.

- Forget to treat for shock if necessary.

- Ignore the injured person's complaints of a headache, dizziness, or sleepiness. Early symptoms can quickly progress.

- Don't keep pushing forward. Often a head injury is a good reason to stop and camp for the night or outright cancel your wilderness plans. Don't keep moving along with hiking or out backing plans, stop and rest.

- Think the person is 'healed' because their symptoms are fading or not getting worse.

Aftercare

Aftercare for head injuries will vary depending on whether it was a concussion or if there was visible physical damage such as a cut or fracture. If there were additional injuries, then it's likely that the injured person will need surgery or extensive medical aid. Most of the time, when the head injury is a mild or moderate concussion, the only option for aftercare is rest. A person who experienced a concussion may needs weeks or months in a low-stress environment with long stretches of rest. They may need to reduce the time they spend at school or work, and even reduce the time spent on hobbies such as watching TV or playing video games.

Additionally, after a head injury, it's advisable that the person lay off, or entirely quit, drinking, or taking any form of drugs. Even caffeine and nicotine affect how the brain operates and can delay its ability to make necessary repairs.

Always seek medical attention after a head injury. Even if you did finish your hiking, fishing, or camping trip, schedule an appointment with your doctor. Everything may seem perfectly fine, but head injuries can lead to brain trauma that may not present themselves for weeks or months. Checking in with a doctor sooner, rather than later, can be a good thing. And, if the injury turns out to be nothing, then you have peace of mind. Head trauma is always tricky and usually requires personalized or individual treatment and aftercare plan.

Chapter 8

Frostbite and Frostnip Injuries

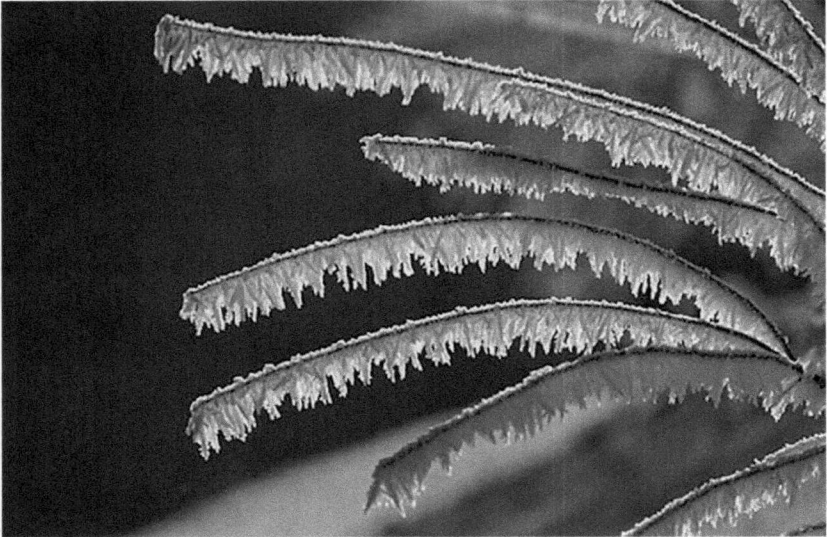

All too often, people underestimate the severe temperatures they may experience when camping, hiking, or even fishing. If you spend a fair amount of time outdoors, you may restrict that time to when the weather is most agreeable. But when planning a long outdoor trip into the wilderness, you may not realize the extreme drop in temperatures that can happen at night, particularly in mountain areas.

For example, while many people are ready to take many precautions in the Blue Ridge Mountains and the Appalachian Mountains that are well-known for drops in temperature, many forget that the west coast Sierra and the Rocky Mountains can be just as treacherous. Frostbite and frostnip injuries can range from very mild to extremely severe. Frostbite may often call for amputation of fingers, noses, and ears. Additionally, detecting frostnip early could deter the development of frostbite entirely.

Frostbite happens because the skin has begun to freeze solid, damaging the tissue beneath on a cellular level. The sensation is that at first, your skin becomes cold and red, which is a sign of frostnip.

Frostnip is a lesser variety of cold injuries, and it doesn't do permanent damage to the skin or the tissue underneath. At the first signs of frostnip, you can begin taking measures to protect the skin and prevent the onset of frostbite. It is a situation where if you fully develop frostbite, you may think back and recognize the moments of frostnip where you could have taken action. Many frostbite victims remark that in hindsight, there was a lot they could have done. Take this cue and take action as soon as you see the signs of frostnip. Even to the point where you see that parts of the skin are turning white or pale, you may be able to save that area of the skin to prevent further frostbite.

It does come in a variety of stages. Frostnip, of course, being the first stage, the second stage being superficial frostbite. Superficial frostbite is what happens when the skin begins to turn white, and the person with the injury report losing sensation in that area. For many, it seems like a relief because the pain of the cold is gone. Afterward and becomes deep frostbite, and you may notice a digit, your nose, your ears, and other more frequently affected areas of the body turn black. When items begin turning black, you can't reverse that damage.

Early symptoms of frostbite include:

- Waxy look to the skin

- Pale skin

- Flakey skin

- Clumsiness from the cold

- Blistering in an attempt to rewarm the area

- Cold and prickling sensations

- Numbness

- Color changes in the skin

One frequent struggle with frostbite is that often people don't realize the frostbite has progressed so severely until another person points it out. If you know that you are spending a good deal of time outdoors, then be sure to constantly evaluate yourself and those in your group for signs of frostnip and frostbite.

How to Determine if this is an Emergency

Frostbite is not an actual emergency because you are at a point where there's nothing that can be done other than amputation. Now, if you have new and unexplained symptoms, then evacuate immediately because you could have more serious cold-related injuries than just frostbite. Additionally, if you have a fever, there's discharge in the frostbitten area, or there's a sudden increase in pain, then evacuate immediately and seek professional medical attention. The primary concern is that frostbite is only a symptom of hypothermia rather than the lone issue that you're handling. Common symptoms of hypothermia can include sleepiness, poor coordination, slurred speech as if the victim was intoxicated, and intense shivering. If none of these symptoms are present, then treat for frostbite as best as possible, and plan on evacuating as weather and travel permit.

There are recommended ways to handle frostnip and the early signs of frostbite.

What to Do with Extreme Cold Injuries

The very first thing that you want to accomplish is to protect the area from any further cold-related damage. If feet are the subject of the frostbite, then do not walk. Walking on a frostbitten foot will likely cause substantial and damage to the tissue far beyond the affected area. If your hands are at the frostbitten stage, then wrap them and try to steadily and slowly warm the tissue. Even when you steadily increase warmth to a frostbitten area, it is possible for blistering to occur within 48 Hours. Those blisters can become a cause for concern if they become infected.

To gradually increase heat to the skin:

- Change to dry or fresh clothing (clothing may not be retaining heat as well as intended or may be sweaty and retaining cold).

- Get out of the wind.

- Seek shelter somewhere you can light a fire.

- Hold hands near, but not over, boiling water or warm water.

- Move the affected area - wiggle toes and fingers.

- Apply aloe vera gel - it's as good for cold-injuries as it is for burns.

- Take ibuprofen for pain management and inflammation.

- Clean and properly cover any opened blisters or cracked skin.

- Stay hydrated - drinking water helps drastically.

- Keep moving to maintain your core temperature.

- Remove all jewelry or wet clothing.

- Dress the area in loose but layered gauze.

A particular issue to note is how to handle frostbitten feet. We already mentioned that people with frostbite on their feet should not be walking on the affected area. Additionally, it is important to remove wet clothing, and it is very likely that the injured person has wet socks and probably wet boots. Removing boots and socks is of particular concern. Remove the boots quickly and get them near a fire to dry. During the time that the boots are drying, the feet may swell. If temperatures and weather were poor enough to cause frostbite, you don't want to attempt to move the person when they can't walk, and they don't have proper foot protection. Ideally, you can remove the boots, and dry them by your fire, change their socks, attempt to regain circulation into the feet, and put the boots back on before the feet swell. That is ideal, but it is not common. For feet, if it is possible to put them in a warm water bath that is circulating, that may substantially change the outcome of their frostbite.

Finally, frostbite is the one instance where medical professionals do recommend aspirating or popping blisters. Only attempt to do this when the blisters are warm; the idea is to prevent fluid from freezing so close to the skin.

What Not to Do with Extreme Cold Injuries

Unfortunately, many of the things that you should not do with an extreme cold injury are exactly what our natural urges want us to do. For example, do not hold your hands over an open flame; direct heat can do more damage to the tissue. Additionally, do not hold a mug or pot filled with near-boiling water, and do not place your hands directly into steam over boiling water. Do not dip the affected area into hot water, although you may temporarily immerse feet and fingers into lukewarm water.

For a complete list:

- Do not rub any of the affected areas.

- Do not keep the area cold, for any reason. Even in the event of injury, don't apply a cold treatment.

- Do not attempt to use rapid rewarming with hot water, steam, or direct application of hot packs.

- Do not allow the area to refreeze. Layer more clothing around the area to protect it and stay in a sheltered place away from cold wind.

Another noteworthy item for this list is to not stay in the area. You may not have anticipated the extreme temperatures, or you may have underestimated the full scale of the local environment. Evacuation is best. If you are in a national or state park, then seek advisement from the rangers. The weather may be abnormal, unexpected, or limited to a specific region of the park. It may be possible to relocate to a different area of the wilderness and not experience the same extreme temperatures.

Aftercare

Aftercare for frostbite is critical when you're coming out of the wilderness. You need professional medical attention, you may need an amputation, you may need surgery, you may need skin grafts, and you will likely need antibiotics. Frostbite often comes with infection; however, it may take a longer period for an infection to set in. If you were coming out of the backcountry with frostbite, then go immediately to an emergency room or emergency medical center. Medical staff there will probably prescribe you an antibiotic, non-steroid a pain reliever such as Tylenol or Ibuprofen, additional pain medication if you are in severe discomfort, and possibly vaccines. Tetanus is an issue that may arise with frostbite, and if you hadn't had a tetanus shot in a while, you would probably get that now.

Chapter 9

Heat Stroke and Dehydration

Heatstroke, sometimes called sunstroke and severe dehydration is often a result of extreme environments and temperatures. Many experienced outdoors people do not head out into hot temperatures without a substantial supply of water or knowledge of where to find fresh, drinkable water in the area. Have a heat stroke and dehydration are still very common injuries. Experiencing heat-related injuries often is not necessarily an emergency, but the symptoms that come with these injuries or illnesses can become life-threatening. Heat exhaustion or heatstroke can lead a person into a coma, make them unresponsive, and raise their core temperature high enough to do brain damage.

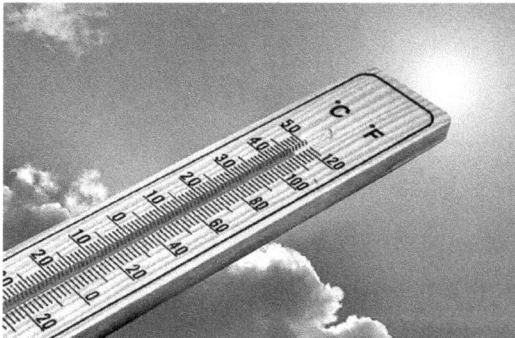

Heatstroke

Heatstroke is the more deadly of the conditions that you can experience in extremely hot temperatures. Heatstroke is life-threatening, but it is preventable. Signs of heatstroke include an elevated heart rate, fast breathing, warm but clammy skin, loss of skin color, irritation, and a body temperature of 104 degrees or higher.

Prior to developing heat stroke, the person will likely experience dehydration and heat exhaustion. Both of these are signs that you should take active steps to prevent heatstroke. Heatstroke is preventable; treat heat exhaustion as quickly as you identify the signs of the condition.

Heatstroke can come with very severe and life-long effects. They may have kidney damage beyond repair, they may lose muscle, and they may lose other vital organ abilities. They may live the rest of their life with impairment and disabilities. You must get emergency help if someone is experiencing heat stroke in the wild. If you have a car nearby, getting them into the car and running the air conditioner can help, but that doesn't excuse them from needing professional intervention.

When help is sought immediately, it's almost guaranteed that they can treat heatstroke successfully with minimal damage to muscle tissue, or organs.

Heat Exhaustion

Heat exhaustion is a milder form of heat illness, although it has many similar symptoms. The primary difference in symptoms between heat exhaustion and heat stroke is that when experiencing heat exhaustion, the person's skin is cool and clammy rather than warm and clammy. They will likely experience a higher heart rate, fast breathing, and they may run a slight fever.

Other signs of heat exhaustion include headache, weakness, tiredness, nausea, and pale skin. However, if you are having trouble differentiating between heat exhaustion and heat stroke, someone with heat exhaustion should have a completely alert mental state and be aware of their environment and what is happening to their body. There should be no signs of agitation or irritation other than standard displeasure at the ambient temperature.

When you are in the later phases of heat exhaustion is a person may become confused, dizzy, experience muscle cramps, and have dark-colored urine. These are signs of salt depletion and will likely progress quickly into heatstroke.

Dehydration

Signs of dehydration typically include a thirst, urinating less often, not urinating at all, not sweating, headaches, dizziness, and changes in skin color. These signs should prompt someone to intake more fluid, and specifically intake fluid with electrolytes. Fluids such as Gatorade, Powerade, and similar drinks are popular among outdoors people because they know it's a quick fix to remedy mild to moderate dehydration. For severe dehydration, electrolytes can dramatically impact the recovery rate.

Some drinks are more capable of rehydrating, and those include water, sports drinks, broth, milk, and all-natural fruit juices. However, you should actively avoid drinking soda, alcohol, and any beverage that includes caffeine, such as coffee, tea, and energy drinks. Drinks with caffeine can cause you to lose fluids more quickly and worsen dehydration.

If you're looking to prepare to fight against dehydration, then you should wear light-colored and loose-fitting clothing. You should also take about one gallon per person per day out into this extreme climate. If you suspect that there will be natural water available, then consider investing in a water filtration device for hikers such as the LifeStraw.

In addition to water filtration devices, you should watch and see where birds are gathering. Birds are a great way to spot water nearby, although carrion birds may not be heading to a watering hole. You can also find water when you see bright green trees. Aspens, willows, cottonwoods, and even palm trees will collect water among their roots. While you don't want to "tap" the tree, you want to dig in toward the roots until you see water pooling.

How to Determine if this is an Emergency

The primary element is that in any case of heat illness, you may need to relocate but not necessarily evacuate. When faced with dehydration, you can probably recover on your own as long as you rest and drink plenty of potable water. Remember that you can always boil natural water to clear it of common bacteria and parasites. If you have no access to water, then retreat to a shaded area and evacuate at night or during the coolest times of the day.

If you, or the person affected, are not showing signs of heatstroke but are merely dehydrated, then you might evaluate your options for resting. Resting, along with water or juice, will often stave off the dehydration, and you can recover. That often means you don't have to evacuate or seek out medical attention. However, if you begin to develop signs of heatstroke, don't hesitate.

If someone is showing signs of heatstroke or more severe signs of heat exhaustion and then evacuate immediately, the longer that a person goes without heat stroke management, the worse the final outcome.

Heatstroke, you can do lasting damage to all of your internal organs, including your brain functioning. If someone appears to be dehydrated, such as having high levels of thirst and showing signs of fatigue, then establish a shaded area or locate a shaded area and rest. This is not an emergency. Signs of heatstroke, such as not being mentally alert or aware of their surroundings, are an emergency and required immediate action.

Heatstroke is the most serious issue to face in regard to heat-related illness. But it is often mistaken. People often believe they're having a heat stroke when they are experiencing heat exhaustion. All the same, evacuation is safer than not evacuating.

What to Do with Heat-Related Illness

Heat-related illness is often believed to only happen in the southwest region of North America. That is not true. While heat-related illness is certainly more rampant through the Great Basin, Mohave, Chihuahuan, and Sonoran deserts, you can experience heat-related illness any time that you're outdoors in moderate to high temperatures. Because of the activity level, you're more likely to become dehydrated quickly in the wilderness. If you're going into a desert, you should have at least one gallon per person, per day. Even with reliable filtration systems, you cannot count on being able to locate water.

If you believe the person has a heat stroke, then evacuate the backcountry immediately.

Now with heat-related injuries, you will want to cool the patient, but not so quickly that it would cause them to shiver. Immediately move the person out of the sun. You can create a shaded area with a tarp and nearby tree or rock. Even a very low to the ground shelter is better than no shelter from the sun. If the person is alert, have them drink water, and fan the body to help bring down their core body temperature. If possible, removing clothing can be helpful, but always considered the immediate environment. Ideally, loose clothing that allows for a lot of airflows will help reduce body temperature and retain the benefits of sweat.

Do avoid moving through the hottest hours during the day. Resting and lying flat along the ground, and also help reduce the effects of heat-related conditions. Resting and lying flat can help bring down the risk of developing heat stroke if someone is currently experiencing heat exhaustion.

What Not to Do with Heat-Related Injuries

Do not ask a person with heat exhaustion, dehydration, or showing signs of heatstroke to continue moving. They need to rest immediately, and they need a shaded area. But you were experiencing dehydration, or heat exhaustion, get yourself to a shaded area or construct a shaded area with minimal effort. If the person you are with or someone in your group is showing signs of heat-related illness, do not ask them to keep going, but instead stopped and created a shaded area.

Do not attempt to lower body temperature with a fever reducer. It won't work.

Additionally, do not try to give someone with heat-related illness symptoms drinks, which may cause further dehydration. Do not give someone with dehydration or heat exhaustion alcohol, caffeinated beverages, or soda. Even if they are complaining of nausea, do not give them Cola syrup, as it can worsen dehydration.

Finally, do not attempt to pour water into the mouth of someone who cannot drink on their own. Their body needs to cool down, and they need to regain mental alertness so that they can sit up and swallow independently.

Don't drink from a cactus. Cactuses are not spiny water bottles. In fact, the fluid inside can blind people, cause burns, and irreparable damage to the esophagus.

Aftercare

Typically, all you can do in the wilderness is an attempt to bring down the person's core body temperature. If that person experienced heat stroke, then medical intervention by professionals is absolutely critical. Doctors will use a variety of approaches to reduce the body's core temperature, including flushing the stomach and rectum with rotations of cold water. They may also redirect a person's blood flow into a collection machine where they can cool the blood and return it to the body.

After you get someone experiencing heat stroke to a medical facility, they will likely need to be treated with anti-seizure and muscle relaxant medications. This person will probably spend a minimum of one to three days in the hospital and may spend more time in a rehabilitation facility. They may need a close team of professionals to work with them to rehabilitate their muscles, and muscle breakdown may not be repairable. Muscle breakdown from the heat and core body temperature can cause damage to the kidneys, and they may be on lifelong treatment for kidney support.

It's important to note here that once you experience heatstroke, you are much more susceptible to heatstroke in the future. If you experienced heatstroke, it doesn't mean that you can't go out into the wilderness. It simply means that you must be more prepared.

Chapter 10

Animal Bites and Related Injuries

A nimal bites are rarely predictable and not often avoidable. While there may be some best practices that you can take when faced with a wild animal, many hikers and campers report that they never even realized the animal was there until they were definitely going to be attacked. Snake bites are rarely seen coming, and small mammals strike with as much speed.

It's important that you carefully treat the bites or scratch correlating to each type of animal. It is not advised to treat a snake bite and a bear scratch the same way. Don't rush, take a moment, and make sure that you're treating the right kind of bite or scratch.

With this information in mind, animal attacks are one of the top fears that backpackers, hikers, and campers share. Animal attacks are not strictly limited to large animals or even what might seem like life-threatening pitches bears, sharks, and sex. Any animal from a bear to a mouse can be a threat. You may not have realized that you stumbled into their home, mismanaged your food, and gave them an easy meal or moved aggressively in some manner.

Snake Bites

Two distinct holes characterize snake bites. You cannot identify the type of snake that bit you based on the bite pattern (unless well experienced in snake bites), but if you are in an area known for a population of venomous snakes, then you should evacuate and seek medical attention. There are 21 different types of venomous snakes in North America, and all are of the viper variety except the coral snake.

To distinguish between the deadly coral snake and the nonvenomous copycat, remember the phrase:

"Black and yellow, kill a fellow. Red and black, venom lack."

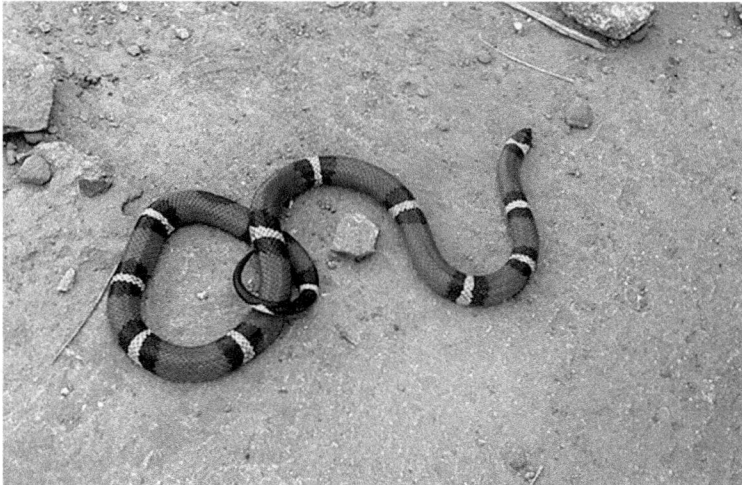

Red and black, venom lack

The phrase is used to distinguish the markings. If the segments of the body are protected within black and yellow bands touching, then it's a coral snake. If the body has a pattern of red and black touching, then it is likely a non-venomous king snake.

Many people wrongfully presume that the southwest is the primary hub of these dangerous creatures, but often deadly snakes are found throughout the South West stretching out to Texas, and all through the South with a high rise of bites in Florida and Alabama. There are even well-known communities of venomous snakes through the Midwest so, if you're bit by a snake, attempt to identify it.

Detecting Venomous Snakes

The venomous snakes in North America are all vipers, which makes identifying them as dangerous or not a bit easier. The most common variety of vipers in North America include rattlesnakes, cottonmouths, copperheads, and diamondbacks; all pit vipers.

Vipers are identifying by:

- Long "hinged" fangs

- Distinctive triangle-shaped head

- Vertically elliptical pupils (two slits going up and down)

- Keeled (rough and slightly raised at the edges) scales

Viper bites are identified by:

- Immediate swelling and pain at the wound site

- Difficulty breathing

- Pain (sometimes only at the wound site, sometimes for the entire limb)

- Vomiting or nausea

- Blurred vision

- Numbness

- Sweating

- Heavy saliva production

- Shock

Mammal Bites and Scratches

From backcountry squirrel bites to bison attacks in Yellowstone, mammals are always something to worry about. The bite itself will vary in look based on the animal, but unlike with snakes, you can often identify the animal with little effort.

Mammal bites will most often happen on the hands, arms, legs, or face. Mammals rarely attack the trunk of the body. Mammals of nearly all sizes can carry hepatitis C, HIV, rabies, and many other bacterial and viral risks.

When it comes to encountering any type of animal in the wild, there is no time for the "warm and fuzzy" moments. Do not approach wild animals, do not feed wild animals,

Large Mammals

Large mammals found throughout North America range from cougars, a moose. Depending on where you are, you may be faced with a wild animal that is double your height. Most large mammals have a prey instinct, and even bison will charge and attack. Many people are lured in with common misconceptions about some of these large creatures. Many people mistakenly believe that moose and bison are gentle or prone to attack, and that could not be further from the truth.

If you are entering territory known for large mammals, especially for aggressive mammals or predators, then ensure that you have proper protection. In addition to an extensive first aid kit, firearms, bear spray, and similar protective equipment are advised.

After a large mammal attack, the bite or scratch itself may have done more physical damage than concern for contracting various bacterial or viral diseases. Although all mammals have the risk of carrying and spreading rabies, if you're faced with a bison, bear, wolf, or other large mammals, you're likely more concerned with the flesh wounds and possible head trauma. Treat open wounds and free bleeding immediately.

Small Mammals

Small mammals can carry all variety of bacteria and viruses. While their bite or scratch may not inherently seem dangerous, the diseases are what is important when camping or hiking near small animals is to manage your food properly. Do not feed wild animals, and do not leave your food in an unprotected area that may attract them. Squirrels, possums, hedgehogs, and more are well-known for chewing or clawing into a bag and opening coolers to get to loose food.

Rabies

All mammals can carry rabies, and almost all rodents do carry rabies. The most common animals to carry rabies in the wild are foxes, bats, skunks, and raccoons. Typically, you don't have to worry about rabies in smaller rodents or larger mammals that don't show signs of the disease.

Infected animals will only transmit rabies after they begin showing clinical signs. For example, it is easy to identify a dog with rabies. If they aren't showing symptoms, the matter may not be urgent. It is still important to seek medical attention, but if you were bitten by an animal that was clearly showing signs of rabies, then seeking medical attention is urgent.

Cases of rabies in humans average about 2 per year in North America. So, take some peace of mind and knowing that it's extremely rare to contract rabies, but don't become complacent because the fox or bat can have rabies and possibly pass it on.

Rabies symptoms can appear anywhere from a few days after the initial bite, two more than a year after the incident. Symptoms may include an itching or tingling feeling, flu-like symptoms, tiredness, fever, and lost appetite. For many people, these are common symptoms for a wide variety of other conditions and diseases.

The trouble is, you cannot wait until symptoms are showing to treat rabies. Once the rabies infection sets in, there's no effective treatment, and very few people have survived rabies.

The course of treatment is a Proactive or preventative approach where you will undergo a series of vaccines over four weeks. It's important to get those vaccines as soon after the bite as possible. Many people will often feel that mammal bites are less concerning than rodent bites or snake bites, especially if it was from a small mammal. Don't underestimate the possibility of rabies. If a mammal bit you, get immediate medical attention to begin the vaccination course as soon as possible.

Rodent and Pest Injuries

Rodent bites happen most frequently among young children, ages five or younger. Regardless of the age, however, rodents almost always strike at hands, feet, ankles, or the face. The trouble isn't the bite itself, which is generally small, shouldn't bleed much, and should heal on its own. However, rats and mice carry rare but extremely deadly types of disease, and other forms of rodents carry harmful diseases as well.

Throughout the greater area of backcountry in North America, rodents run freely and have a widespread reign over territory. From Florida to Kansas, you can bet that field mice, chipmunks, gophers, rats, and lemmings, all of which can bring on some injury.

Rodents can carry the following well-known diseases:

- Rabies

- "Rat-bite" fever

- Rat tapeworm

- Salmonellosis

- Asthma

- Hantavirus

- Toxoplasmosis

- Trench fever

- Typhoid

- Typhus

- Well's Disease

People often forget or completely mistake the damages that come from rodents and are close relatives of squirrels. Throughout the Southwest in North America, rodents are among the most hazardous and destructive to people. That's often associated with the damage they can do in a home and the dangers of being around the animals' waste.

A bite from a rodent, squirrel, and other common pests can call for a less urgent evacuation. If a rodent bit you, know that your body may be subject to extremely rare, but fatal diseases. Often, doctors are not sure how to proceed with treatment unless they have the animal and can test it. In the backcountry, that's highly unlikely, and you may have to undergo treatment for a variety of diseases whether you contracted them or not.

Risks of Hantavirus and Plague

The two most pressing concerns that come with rodent bites are hantavirus and plague. While these two are ever-present, and people who work in construction or service industries are well aware of the risks, most people aren't. Even experienced hikers and backpackers are not familiar with the risks of rodent-carried diseases.

Rats and mice specifically carry the plague, while most people associate them with the bubonic plague, they can carry three different types of plague. The United States averages between 1 and 17 cases of human plague per year, almost all associated with a rat, mouse, or flea bite.

More concerning, and more common is the hantavirus that seemed to come from rat and mouse bites. Hantavirus is more present in mice than it is in rats, and it can be contracted not just from a bite, but from coming into close contact with rodent waste.

Hantavirus has a high fatality rate, and it is the most common reason why people do need to evacuate after a mouse bite. You know the hantavirus is most common among deer mice, which are widespread across North America. If you suspect that one of those cute little brown fluffy mice is the one that bit you, then plan on making a doctor's appointment when you get back to civilization. Symptoms of plague and hantavirus can take days or weeks to appear.

How to Determine if this is an Emergency

Some snake bites do not require medical care or intervention if you can be certain that the snake was non-venomous. If you suspect the snake was venomous or could be venomous, evacuate immediately. If possible, call the nearest medical center and inform them of the snake bite, suspected type of snake, and that you're coming in. Not all medical centers carry antivenom, and they may need to have it brought into their center.

Nearly all mammals or rodents will require medical attention because of the high risk of contracting extremely dangerous diseases. Any mammal that has a high probability of rabies requires immediate evacuation, as any delay in treatment for rabies could be fatal.

If you are fairly certain, there is no risk for rabies. Then you may delay seeking treatment if the wound is controllable. If the wound is visibly significant, then do not delay, evacuate immediately.

The degree of emergency after an animal bite or animal attack depends not only on the animal but on the damage experience. Because of the diseases that mammals and rodents can carry, it is often advised to seek medical attention quickly even if the bite seems under control and there is minimal damage. Many backpackers and hikers do not immediately evacuate if the animal bite is controllable, the bleeding slows or stops quickly, and the bite or scratch can be handled as a standard flesh wound.

Keep in mind with the snake bites, if you can, without doubt, identify that the snake is non-venomous, then there's likely no need for evacuation. If you know that the snake is of a non-venomous variety, then treat it as a standard flush food.

What to Do with Animal-Related Injuries

animal-related injuries and must be treated differently pertaining to what type of animal it is. There are various do's and don'ts that come with each animal variety pertaining to the categories of snakes, mammals, and rodents, or common pests. All are exceptionally common throughout North America, and when you're in the backcountry or wilderness, you're in their domain. Most animals attack as a measure of defense or self-protection, while predators may attack to establish dominance or view you as prey.

It is imperative to remain aware of your surroundings at all times and observe early warning signs of attack.

Snakes may rattle or hiss to make you aware of their presence, and except for the coral snake, will likely not attack unless provoked. If you are in an area where venomous snakes are common, be very aware of where these snakes reside. For example, most cottonmouth bites happen because people are not aware that they are stepping on top of leaves where cottonmouths had made their home.

Most large mammals will make their presence known with a cry or changing stance. For example, a bear rearing up and standing on its hind legs is the warning of an impending attack. If you have proper protective equipment such as bear spray, that is your opportunity to use it.

Many small mammals will attack to obtain food or to defend their presence. Common instances of small mammal attacks include setting up camp or putting up a tent, over gopher networks, or where possums have nested. With small mammals, there is rarely a sign of attack, or acknowledgment that they are present.

What to Do with Venomous Snake Bites

After identifying whether the snake is venomous, or potentially venomous, you'll want' to initiate treatment. Depending on the type of snake, the location of the bite, and the dose of venom, the bitten person may have minutes or days to live if they do not receive treatment.

For a venomous snake bite:

1. Note the time of the bite.

2. If possible, note the type of snake.

3. Call 911, or evacuate immediately for the nearest medical facility.

4. Stay calm, and still, if possible - movement can quicken the travel of the venom.

5. Remove jewelry or constrictive clothing as swelling will be immediate.

Nonvenomous bites treat as any other flesh wound but do not administer a cold compress or raise the bite area over the heart. Watch for signs of infection.

For a mammal bite or scratch:

1. Stop the bleeding

2. Wash the area thoroughly with mild soap

3. Use antibiotic cream or gel.

4. Cover the wound with dry and clean gauze or material

5. Keep the wound area elevated.

Contact a medical professional if there are signs of infection within two days. If the animal is a high-risk rabies carrier such as a bat or a fox, then seek immediate medical attention.

For a rodent bite:

1. Wash the area with mild soap and warm water

2. Dry with a clean towel or gauze

3. Apply antibiotic ointment

4. Cover with a bandage

Seek medical attention with ease. Symptoms of diseases carried by rodents may take days or weeks to appear.

What Not to Do with Animal-Related Injuries

Do not assume that everything is fine when the bleeding stops. Also, do not assume that after the bite that the animal has vacated the area.

What not to do with snakebites (venomous or non-venomous):

1. Do not use a tourniquet.

2. Do not provide any medication.

3. Do not raise the wound over the person's heart.

4. Do not attempt to use any type of suction device, or "suck" the venom out with your mouth.

5. Do not use a cold compress.

6. Do not cut into the bite area.

These are common snakebite first aid myths that have all been proven as ineffective or with the potential to cause more harm.

Generally, mammal bites and rodent bites can be treated as flesh wounds with standard cleaning, antibiotic gel, and wrapping. However, the concern here does not wane if it is only a small bite. Small bites can carry substantial diseases, and you must respond appropriately.

Aftercare

Aftercare for animal bites will vary depending on the severity of the bite. If the bite was small, and minimal bleeding, and was able to receive cleaning and a fresh wrap immediately, then check in with your doctor when you get out of the wilderness.

If the bite was deep or similar to a puncture wound, then you will likely need to follow up with your primary care physician to ensure that there is not extensive damage to the muscle or tissue.

In the event of an animal that is known for carrying rabies, such as most mammals, bats, foxes, and rats, then you may have to undergo a week of ongoing vaccinations to ward off or protect you from rabies. Additionally, if you're bitten by common disease-carrying animals such as mice or squirrels, then you may have to undergo additional vaccinations for various other diseases.

When it comes to more extreme animal bites and attacks, you may spend days, weeks, or months in a hospital or rehabilitation facility. Large mammals can do extensive damage in a very short amount of time, but many people have unexpected survival stories. The aftercare in extreme animal attacks often includes treatment for possible diseases contracted from the animal, treatment for broken bones, muscle damage, tissue damage, nerve damage, and drama, and more. Rehabilitation may take years, and victims of severe animal attacks may never fully recover strength, range of motion, and use of limbs.

Chapter 11

Illness and Allergic Reactions in the Wild

Sustaining illnesses or allergic reactions in the wild is, at best, a traumatic experience. Illnesses can come on from eating unsafe foods or improperly prepared food. Additionally, allergic reactions can come from skin contact or ingesting items that you may or may not have known you had an allergy to. Severe allergic reactions can happen not only from food but from contact with various plants and even tree bark or dust. Allergic reactions and illnesses can be life-threatening; someone experiencing anaphylactic shock may only have a minuscule time frame to receive professional medical attention. Someone experiencing illness in the wild may experience dehydration or organs shut down if they don't receive proper medical care.

Eating the Wrong Thing or Improperly Preparing Food in the Wild

Various hikers, fishers, backpackers, and campers have found themselves in the full throes of food poisoning on what should have been a vacation. Getting poisoning at camp is far more common than many people believe. Food poisoning can come from eating the wrong thing, poor foraging technique, and improperly preparing food. The good news is that most instances of food poisoning get better on their own with rest and hydration. The primary concern is that in the backcountry, you may not have access to potable water or easy access to peaceful rest.

In regard to foraging, mushroom poisoning will attack the nervous system and can result in death. Signs of mushroom poisoning include shrunken pupils, heavy saliva production, foaming or frothing-at-the-mouth, vertigo. Mushroom poisoning will attack the nervous system and can result in death. Signs of mushroom poisoning include shrunken pupils, heavy saliva production, foaming or frothing at the mouth, vertigo, coma, and seizures.

Basic guidelines for foraging to help prevent you from eating the wrong thing include not eating anything you can't identify, and don't eat anything that might be venomous or has a stinger. Generally speaking, stay away from plants unless you know you can undoubtedly identify what you're foraging, and have a guide book on edible plants available.

If you do fall prey to food illness and the wild, then focus on handling the symptoms. Trying to move around or trying to evacuate may waste valuable energy that you need to recover. Most food poisoning can recover on its own unless you ingest something deadly.

How to Handle Nausea, Vomiting, and Diarrhea

Almost every form of food poisoning will result in diarrhea, nausea, and vomiting. Other symptoms often include headache, lethargy, fever, and cold sweat. You can treat all of these symptoms as long as you have access to drinking water.

The most commonly experienced complication that comes with food poisoning is dehydration. The quick rate of bodily fluids leaving your body causes you to lose not only liquids, but sodium, potassium, and other necessary electrolytes. Symptoms of food poisoning can show up between six and 48 hours after ingestion and can last for 48 hours to several weeks.

When handling these primary symptoms, try to avoid solid foods. Instead, choose soft or easy to digest foods such as crackers, bread, bananas, or rice. When camping or hiking, it's always smart to keep a pack of saltine crackers around. If you plan on foraging or hunting the entire time you are in the wilderness, then avoid eating plants and instead opt for insect life. Be sure to avoid anything venomous, which means staying away from furry bugs (bees), brightly colored (centipedes), or have more than six legs (spiders and millipedes).

You may have anti-diarrhea medication, which can come with some side-effects but may also help prevent you from losing fluids at a vital level.

Ensure that you have plenty of drinkable water on hand. If you did not bring enough water for the length of time that you will likely be sick, boil fresh water. Or, have someone at your camp boil or filter water for you. Boiling water will remove most of the biological contaminants but will not filter out naturally present minerals or metals such as lead or iron. After boiling, freshwater is safe to drink. If you have salt and sugar, you can add one teaspoon of salt with four teaspoons of sugar to 1 liter of water.

Poisoning

Poisoning can happen in the wilderness, and the most common elements of poisoning include mushrooms, white gas, and carbon monoxide. Each of these types of poisoning can be fatal, but all can easily be treated. Additionally, although many people worry about the presence of children in camps or when hiking, the most common poisoning accidents happen to adults. A lot of it is complacency or believing that they were safely making camp more comfortable.

Mushroom poisoning is among the most common in adults between teen and young-adult years. Evidently, people are trying to add a hallucinogenic effect to their dinner in the outdoors. Children, however, are the most frequent consumers of wild-growing or natural mushrooms, and often have no problem with poisoning. When adults go looking for mushrooms that they believe will have a hallucinogenic effect, they often pick the most poisonous mushrooms because of distinct colors, spots, and suspicious shapes.

Generally, you should avoid eating natural mushrooms or mushrooms found in the wild. If you suspect that someone has consumed a poisonous mushroom, treat immediately. Treatment for potentially ingesting poisonous mushrooms is one of the very few times where vomiting is recommended. Induce vomiting, or if you have activated charcoal, then bind the toxin with the charcoal. Vomiting will only be effective if they can induce vomiting within an hour of ingestion. If at all possible, attempt to induce vomiting naturally rather than using ipecac or a similar vomit inducer. Vomit induced through epic at or vomit inducers are often very forceful and can result in trauma to the esophagus as well as injury. If you cannot manually induce vomiting and do not have ipecac, you can mix two tablespoons of mild soap with a very small amount of water.

You mustn't induce vomiting if the person is not conscious or has disorders that can result in seizures.

White gas poisoning is common when hikers, backpackers, and outdoors people accidentally take a drink out of their fuel bottle instead of their water bottle. Often these people are completely fine as long as they didn't accidentally inhale any of the gas. Getting white gas in your lungs can be deadly and cause deadly cases of pneumonia. If you inhaled white gas, evacuate immediately. If you only swallowed the gas, then you want to dilute it as much as possible. Dilute the gas by drinking water. But if you have powdered milk, then mix up a batch and drink that. Take some time to rest until you feel better.

Carbon monoxide poisoning is common among people who choose to cook in their tents rather than outdoors. If you're in a particularly cold or windy area, it's better to have ready-to-eat food or try to cook outside. Carbon monoxide poisoning often happens because it's inhaled, and people normally have no idea. It is one of the most serious and common poison threats in the wild, but the treatment is simple.

The early symptoms of carbon monoxide poisoning include headache, vomiting, poor coordination, irritability, poor judgment, confusion, and nausea. If you experience these and do not take action, the next step is coma and then death. Death usually occurs because of heart failure as the carbon monoxide poisoning changes the flow and behavior of your red blood cells.

The treatment? Get fresh air. If someone is irritable or showing early signs of carbon monoxide poisoning, then get outside. Fresh air over time will completely reverse the symptoms of carbon monoxide poisoning. But if you experienced high levels of carbon monoxide poisoning, then you may need supplemental oxygen or a high-pressure chamber.

When to Evacuate Due to Abdominal Pain

In most situations, abdominal pain is a symptom of a generalized illness or possible injury. A parasite will present ten days or more of diarrhea along with fatigue, and foul-smelling stool or gas. The best you can do in those situations is to treat diarrhea by attempting to stay hydrated and evacuating when possible.

Stomach aches are generally not life-threatening and are characterized by cramping that comes and goes. If cramping is persistent or relentless, then evacuate immediately.

If the person presents a fever over a hundred and two degrees, chills lasting more than 12 hours, consistent or constant pain lasting for more than 12 hours, blood in their vomit or waste, or goes into shock, then evacuate immediately for urgent medical attention.

Allergic Reactions to Poison Oak and Poison Ivy

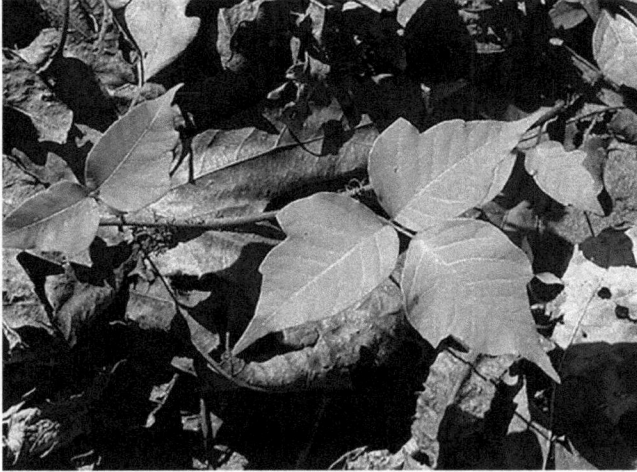

Touching any part of the poison ivy or poison oak plant will cause an instant reaction, including swollen skin, severe itching, blisters, and a persistent rash.

Treating poison oak or poison ivy, it calls for immediate cleansing or deep cleaning of the area with soap and water. The idea is to prevent the oil binding to the skin. The longer that oil sets on the skin, the deeper its roots.

After you wash the skin, then apply a cold compress, and if you have antihistamines available to take them. An antihistamine such as Benadryl can drastically relieve the itching. A bacterial infection is not likely, but it can occur, and inhalation of burning poison ivy or poison oak can be fatal.

If you come across poison ivy or poison oak, likely, you don't need to evacuate, although you might choose to do so for your own comfort. The fact of the matter here is that you're going to have a very uncomfortable two to 18 days while you recover. There is very little you can do. Even at home, the best approach to cooling the itch is an oatmeal bath, which is often seen as ineffective.

Mild Allergic Reactions

Mild allergic reactions are extremely common both in the wilderness and in most households. Allergic reactions can come from a bee sting, mosquito bite, brushing up against a plant that doesn't sit well with your body, or even something and having a mild allergy. You don't need to rush off if you develop a hive or are a little itchy. But you should carefully monitor the extent of your allergy. Mild allergic reactions are not likely to progress, but when they do, it may lead to anaphylactic shock.

With mild allergies, you can treat them with an over-the-counter antihistamine such as Benadryl, or you can grin and bear it. If you don't have Benadryl or a similar antihistamine, then you may zero options available to you for treating the allergic reaction.

For skin reactions, you can curb some of the itches with a cold compress. Make sure that you don't directly expose skin to ice, though. Although ice is a great way to soothe an itch, it can do quite a bit of damage and even lead to unintended frostbite.

Another way to stay comfortable during allergic reactions is to stay hydrated. Miraculously, drinking water can help your body appropriately respond to the mild reaction, and ease a lot of the symptoms such as hives and swelling.

Severe Allergic Reactions

Many people have general allergies, which may result in some skin irritation, hives, and general itchiness. But large percentages of the population also experienced severe allergic reactions to particular elements, foods, and substances. You can be allergic to almost anything that you would encounter in the wilderness, and if you don't know that you had an injury, you may be drastically unprepared. If you begin to have an immune response to a foreign substance or a substance that you know you're allergic to, then you need to take immediate action. That immediate action may not always call for evacuation of the area. In some situations, if you're more than a few hours away from a medical facility, then evacuation may not be a lifesaving maneuver.

Epinephrine

An epi-pen or similar form of epinephrine is the go-to solution for severe allergic reactions that obstruct the airway or possible anaphylactic shock.

Anaphylactic shock is a life-threatening issue and requires epinephrine. You cannot treat anaphylaxis without medication.

If someone experiences a severe allergic reaction and epinephrine is not available, proceed with the following steps.

Lay Back with Feet Elevated

Anaphylaxis demands the person stay calm, and it's best to do that with a person lying on their back. Help them lay down and try to keep them as calm as possible. Raise their feet by about a foot and then cover them with a blanket. You'll notice that this slightly deviates from standard shock treatment.

Remove Tight Fitting Items

Whether it is jewelry or clothing, remove any tight-fitting item. Not only can this restrict breathing, but it can cause discomfort and panic if they begin to swell and feel that tightness.

Vomiting and Bleeding

If the person begins vomiting or bleeding, turn them on their side. Vomiting is not often common with anaphylaxis, but bleeding can be. Often these days and times are alarming, so it's important to avoid panic. Often these symptoms are alarming, so it's important to avoid panic. Bleeding and vomiting may be a sign that the allergy is reaching its peak. However, it may also be a sign that the reaction is worsening.

Perform CPR or Rescue Breathing

If a person stops breathing or becomes unresponsive, then initiate CPR or rescue breathing immediately. When giving CPR for anaphylactic shock, you want to do hands-only CPR. That means compressions only without rescue breathing. If the person loses all signs of life, initiate rescue breathing with chest compressions. Keep in mind that you need to do 100 compressions per minute and, if possible, to get help on the scene.

Evacuate or Contact a Local Authority for EMS Support

If someone is clearly entering anaphylactic shock, cannot breathe, and the allergic reaction is not getting better, then evacuate immediately. There are times with anaphylaxis that the symptoms and body response can be fatal within minutes. Even when people are at home and nearby medical facilities, it's possible to not get medical help in time.

Contacting a nearby medical facility can help reduce the damage done from anaphylaxis and possibly save their life. An emergency medical response team may be able to come to your location or meet you nearby and deliver lifesaving epinephrine.

Chapter 12

Quick Reference
for Medical Procedures

Throughout this book, there are brief instructions for medical procedures that may be lifesaving. This chapter is dedicated to a quick reference with detailed explanations into how to apply specific practices or techniques correctly. Some of these are present in other areas of the book where they are most pertinent. However, a quick reference is vital for anyone who needs immediate instructions and knows the appropriate procedure to treat the injury. Please keep in mind that all of these should be accompanied with professional training and certification. If you're an avid outdoors person, then you should consider going through an extensive first aid course, or Red Cross certification.

While certifications are not necessary to administer lifesaving action, there is always the risk of performing a procedure or technique improperly. We are not responsible for any improperly performed or applied procedures or medical techniques.

Procedures and Courses that Can Save Lives

With each of the procedures below, we've also included where you can find courses to get proper certification for the procedure or technique. If you're reading ahead of time, then plan out when you can attend a class. If you are currently in an emergency, then follow the procedure to the best of your ability.

Remember to follow basic safety courses during every procedure:

- Wear latex gloves
- Check the ABCs (Airway, Breathing, Circulatory system or blood flow)
- Survey the person for possible neck or spine injuries before moving them.
- Check your surroundings for immediate dangers.

CPR and Rescue Breathing

CPR can come in two forms, with rescue breathing, and without rescue breathing. Without breaths, CPR may also be called hands-only CPR40. Always start by assessing the scene and determining why they need CPR. There are times to use hand-only CPR and then times to use full CPR with rescue breathing.

Use hands-only when:

- Suspected cardiac arrest
- Sudden collapse in a teen or adult
- Becoming unresponsive during choking.

Use hands and rescue breathing when:

- Performing CPR after near-drowning

- Overdose

- Poisoning

- Severe asthma attack

Step One:

Lay the person flat on their back and straighten their neck. Tilt the forehead back with a palm, and then use your index and middle finger to guide the chin into a lifted but natural position. Open the mouth slightly.

Step Two:

Listen for breathing carefully.

Step Three:

Push hard and fast. Place one hand on top of the other. Curl the fingers of the top hand around the bottom hand, hold the fingers of the bottom hand upward. Place hands in the middle of the chest and press down at least 2-inches deep into the chest. Do this at a pace of 100 - 120 compressions per minute.

Step Four:

Tightly close your thumb and forefinger around the meaty areas of the nostrils. Seal your mouth over theirs and blow deeply for two seconds. For infants, blow gently for one second and only perform compressions with two fingers from one hand over the chest bone just below the nipple line.

Give one breath every six seconds.

Continue until:

- The person begins breathing on their own

- An AED (and someone knowledgeable of using an AED) is available.

- EMS arrives

- You can no longer perform CPR due to exhaustion.

- The area has become unsafe for you and/or the injured person.

Broken ribs are common in administering CPR and appear in about 40% to 70% of CPR cases. Additional injuries are especially common in children and the elderly. Although

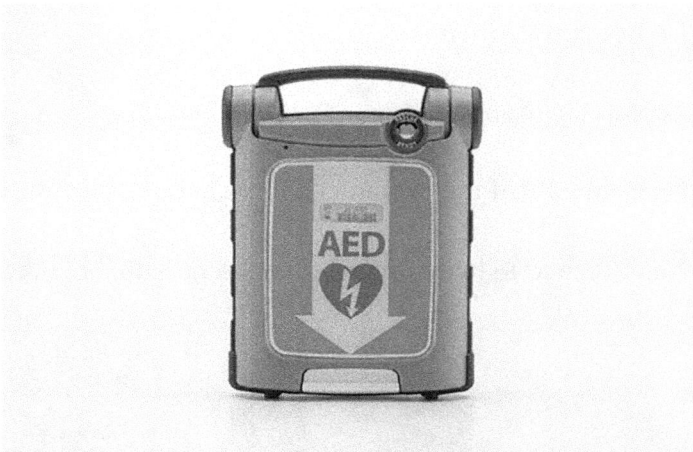

Treating for Shock

Treating for shock is very straightforward but only actually effective if you identify the early signs of shock. Either way, follow one of two procedures.

If the person is responsive:

1. Lay them flat on their back.

2. Elevate their feet by six to eight inches.

3. If not related to heat illness, cover them with a blanket.

4. Attempt to keep the person still.

5. Watch for progression or regression of symptoms.

If the person is not responsive:

1. Lay the person on their side; if there are neck injuries, do not move them.

2. Do not elevate their feet.

3. Loosen any tight clothing.

4. Perform CPR if the person is not breathing

5. If not related to heat illness, cover them with a blanket.

When treating for shock, also make sure that you don't permit the person to eat anything, and if it's not related to any heat illness, don't allow them to drink anything until they've recovered.

How to Use a Tourniquet

Using a tourniquet requires more force than most people feel comfortable exerting. Because of the force required, you will need a strip of cloth or fabric and a straight object that is at least eight inches long because it's not a tourniquet if you don't have a windlass.

1. Cut a strip of fabric or rip a relatively clean shirt to full length.

    *   Fabric should be a minimum of 2 or 3-inches wide to compress arteries and veins.

2. Wrap the material between two and four inches above the wound, closer to the torso. Only wrap the material along sections of the body that only have one bone, such as the thigh or upper arm.

3. Tie a secure knot.

4. Lay the "twist stick" or similar item across the knot.

5. Tie another, very secure, knot over the twist stick.

6. Use the twist stick to tighten the tourniquet.

It is important to note with a tourniquet that doing it incorrectly can cause severe damage and even further complicate the blood loss. If the blood loss is not stopped, it can lead to life-threatening complications quickly. Many people don't properly apply a tourniquet because they are afraid of hurting the injured person, but the pain should not be a factor. It is extremely unlikely that you will break the bone or cause more injury by tightening a tourniquet. To ease some pain when tightening the tourniquet with the windlass, you can always slightly raise the windlass when twisting it.

What to Expect from First Aid Training

In first aid training either through local first aid programs, hospital first aid training programs, or the Red Cross Association, you should learn all of the techniques here except possibly how to use a tourniquet.

Most first aid and CPR training will include:

- CPR, compressions, and rescue breathing.

- Recognizing emergencies

- Deciding how to act in an emergency

- Key factors in treatment and emergency response

- How to respond to an unconscious or unresponsive adult

- How to respond to an unconscious or unresponsive child or infant

- Working an AED or Automated External Defibrillator

- How to respond to choking

- Recovery Position

- Bandaging flesh wounds

- Splints

The trouble that many people face is that the first aid training can tell them exactly what to do, but not to prepare for facing the injury head-on. Many people will feel a moment of panic, but remember your training and begin by assessing the situation. Keep in mind that your training gave you all the knowledge necessary to handle the most common injuries experienced at home, and many of those are similar or exactly the same to injuries in the wild. The only mild difference is that you may need to be more creative with your available resources. Limited resources are a common obstacle for outdoorsy people, and you must evaluate what you have on hand and use the best substitute materials available.

It is highly likely that you will need material or fabric, and for that, you can often use a clean or fresh shirt or towel. Also, be prepared to resource branches, sticks, and other wood materials for twist sticks for tourniquets, or for bracing a splint.

Understanding Evacuation and Evacuation Levels

Evacuation levels were not discussed at great length in the various sections but only addressed when evacuation may be necessary. There are different methods of evacuation, but most depend on the resources and number of people available. Self-evacuation is common among sensationalized survival stories. But evacuation can also occur with assistance, a simple carry, construction of a leader, and even a vehicle if it's available. In most cases, seal the treatment, or wilderness treatment can definitely handle non-life-threatening injuries. Rapid evacuation may not be necessary in the majority of cases. But there are times where the medical window to treat life-threatening injuries or illnesses can be within hours or even minutes. Here is a quick overview of evacuation levels to help guide you in understanding how urgently you may need to evacuate the wilderness.

Level One

A level 1 evacuation is required when the patient is in immediate danger, and their injury or illness may result in death. A level 1 evacuation is most common for people experiencing ICP, extreme shock, respiratory distress, hypothermia, and cardiac arrest. A level 1 evacuation is also necessary when the person experiences a snake bite from a venomous snake.

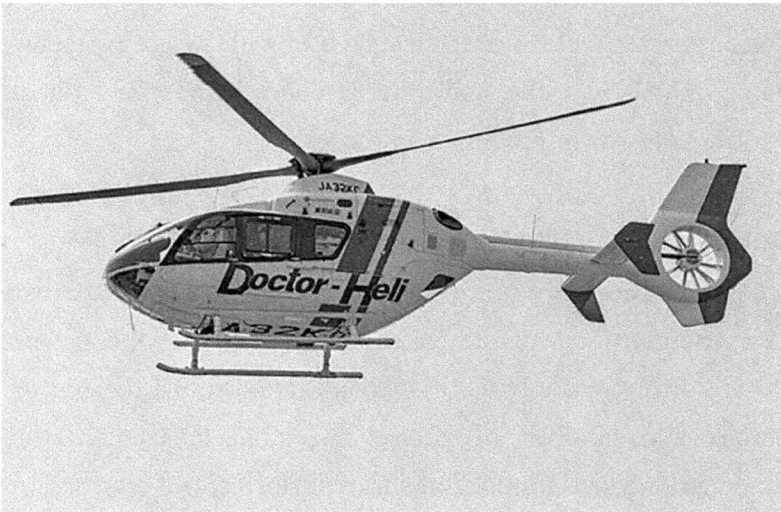

Level Two

Level 2 evacuation is when the injury or illness has the potential to become life-threatening. Damage to the spine or spinal cord, near-drowning, severe concussions, and some types of head trauma will call for a level 2 evacuation. These evacuations also include responses to heatstroke. The situation here is that you want to evacuate but need to take precautions to protect the patient. At this point, you can take greater action to protect the health and welfare of the person by taking the time to evacuate safely. The matter is urgent, but you may need to construct a litter, create splints, or similar to protect the injured person.

Level Three

Level 3 is officially a non-urgent evacuation. It means that the injury or illness is not always threatening and has very little potential to become life-threatening. In these cases, the person who experienced the injury should be able to resume normal activity in just a few hours. For example, if they received the concussion, and within a few hours can't sit up, eat, and normally communicate, then it would call for a level 3 evacuation. Level three evacuations are common with moderate to low-grade concussions, flesh wounds, and dislocations.

Level Four

At level 4, there is no evacuation necessary. It means that the person who was injured is not facing any life-threatening concerns or issues. The wilderness treatment may have been a complete success, and they should be able to go through all normal activities. The patient may have experienced minor wounds, flesh wounds, environmental injuries, moderate degrees of dehydration, and similar.

Experiencing a sprain, or small amount of food poisoning in the wilderness often calls for a level 4 evacuation. These are instances where seeking medical attention may not only be unnecessary but may serve no purpose. For example, going to an emergency room for a sprained will likely result in an emergency room staff, sending you home asking you to schedule an appointment with your standard practitioner.

Always Be Aware and Vigilant

When you're outdoors, it's important always to be very aware of your surroundings and possible dangers. What is arguably more important though is to be aware of all elements of an injury before beginning treatment. Always take time to survey the injured person, and if you're treating yourself, then be sure to evaluate your physical state carefully to observe all possible injuries. Often, people don't realize that there were additional injuries until much later, and that mistake can be life-threatening or life-changing.

You should always be on the lookout for additional injuries, dangers, or developing issues related to the injury during treatment and recovery.

Infection can start with bites, flesh wounds, blisters from both cold and heat-related wounds, and even from near-drowning. Always survey for signs of infection, including an increase in heart rate, fever, and disorientation.

For injuries relating to head trauma, you need to always be on the lookout for ICP and to ensure that concussions aren't worsening. There are always ways to remedy an injury partially, but there are times when you can't do anything to stop some events. If ICP, secondary drowning, or severe heatstroke set in, then there is typically nothing that can be done in the wilderness. These conditions or injuries may be so severe that even professional medical intervention wouldn't guarantee the health or life of the injured person.

If, for any reason, you believe that the person needs immediate medical intervention, go with your gut, and evacuate. However, always take care that you evacuate safely. Remember that some injuries may make it unrealistic for the injured person to walk out on their own. They may need extensive support, splints, or may change how long it takes to get to civilization.

It's always best to take precautions or the safer route. Use the procedures and techniques to the best of your ability, and if you are not confident that you can perform the procedure correctly, then see if another person can. If not, you may be the only person available to perform a potentially lifesaving technique or procedure. Follow the best advice possible or seek out immediate professional medical intervention. If you are more than 24 hours away from nearby medical treatment, then you should have the appropriate resources or knowledge to perform these types of procedures. If not, then at least have the contact information for nearby authorities and medical centers.

Conclusion

A fter referencing specific chapters as needed or reading through the entirety of the book, you should thoroughly understand how to gauge an emergency and how to respond quickly. Many injuries in the wilderness will call for some level of evacuation, but not every injury calls for immediate evacuation. You must always use your best judgment to assess the injuries and the situation. This book is a good resource material to have saved onto your phone directly so you can reference it quickly, whether you have service or not. You can quickly flip to the chapter that addresses the immediate or current injury.

You should fully understand how to evacuate the wilderness and how to do so safely in addition to treating various injuries and illnesses in the wild. Additionally, you should have obtained the full knowledge not to take evacuation lightly, but always keep in mind that there will be times when you cannot do anything for the injured person in the wild.

This book should provide a comprehensive guide to the most common injuries that people experience in the outdoors, whether they're boating, hiking, camping, or immersing themselves in nature.

Keep in mind that proper preparation and a calm approach to treating injuries can substantially change your outdoor experience. Be prepared, and enjoy the great wilderness!

References

https://blog.scoutingmagazine.org/2017/05/08/be-prepared-scout-motto-origin

https://wikem.org/wiki/wilderness_preparedness

https://www.adc-fl.com/locations/mount-dora/building-an-outdoors-first-aid-kit

https://www.wta.org/go-outside/trail-smarts/like-your-life-depends-on-it-building-your-first-aid-kit

https://www.webmd.com/first-aid/does-this-cut-need-stitches

https://www.outdoors.org/articles/amc-outdoors/how-to-treat-cuts-wounds-on-the-trail

http://www.alertdiver.com/wilderness_Wound_Care

https://medlineplus.gov/ency/article/000043.htm

https://kidshealth.org/en/teens/cuts.html

http://www.childrenshospital.org/conditions-and-treatments/conditions/s/sprains-and-strains

https://www.webmd.com/first-aid/understanding-sprains-strains-treatment

https://www.tgomagazine.co.uk/skills/first-aid-how-to-treat-sprains-and-strains/

https://villageec.com/blog/when-to-go-to-the-er-for-a-sprained-ankle/

https://www.mayoclinic.org/diseases-conditions/sprained-ankle/diagnosis-treatment/drc-20353231

https://www.scoi.com/patient-resources/education/articles/should-you-ice-or-heat-injury

https://www.medicinenet.com/drowning/article.htm

https://www.pfizer.com/news/featured_stories/featured_stories_detail/how_to_tell_if_someone_is_drowning

https://www.mountsinai.org/health-library/injury/near-drowning

https://www.wildmedcenter.com/blog/drowning

https://www.saintlukeskc.org/health-library/first-aid-rescue-breathing

https://www.healthline.com/health/dry-drowning#takeaway

https://www.mana.md/should-i-worry-about-dry-drowning-and-secondary-drowning

https://www.readersdigest.ca/health/conditions/essential-cpr-steps/

https://ameriburn.org/who-we-are/media/burn-incidence-fact-sheet/

https://www.theoutbound.com/hartley-brody/how-to-treat-the-6-most-common-injuries-in-the-backcountry

https://www.cdc.gov/masstrauma/factsheets/public/burns.pdf

https://stanfordhealthcare.org/medical-conditions/skin-hair-and-nails/burns/

https://www.webmd.com/pain-management/guide/pain-caused-by-burns

https://www.wildernessarena.com/skills/first-aid-health-and-first-aid/preventing-and-treating-shock

https://www.mayoclinic.org/first-aid/first-aid-shock/basics/art-20056620

https://blog.nols.edu/2015/09/04/treating-burns-in-the-backcountry

https://www.mayoclinic.org/first-aid/first-aid-burns/basics/art-20056649

https://advancedtissue.com/2015/06/6-mistakes-to-avoid-with-burn-wounds/

https://www.healthline.com/health/home-remedies-for-burns#see-a-doctor

https://www.qvh.nhs.uk/wp-content/uploads/2015/09/A-guide-to-burns-aftercare-v1-Rvw-Sept-2013.pdf

https://www.nhs.uk/common-health-questions/accidents-first-aid-and-treatments/how-do-i-know-if-i-have-broken-a-bone/

https://medlineplus.gov/ency/article/000014.htm

http://www.theoutdoorsurvivalguide.com/fractures.html

https://www.coloradowm.org/blog/blog/splinting-review/

https://www.wilderness-survival.net/medicine-4.php

https://www.healthline.com/health/how-to-pop-your-shoulder#after-it-happens

https://www.deseret.com/1995/5/14/19175266/putting-dislocated-kneecap-back-in-place-is-best-course-in-wilds

https://www.youtube.com/watch?v=MAKqZZrzdOE

https://www.youtube.com/watch?v=ANA2b-g3qaw

https://www.wemjournal.org/article/S1080-6032(08)70163-7/pdf

https://www.latinaproject.com/tbi/coup.html

https://gla-rehab.com/impact-of-mild-traumatic-brain-injury-and-how-to-treat/

https://gla-rehab.com/impact-of-mild-traumatic-brain-injury-and-how-to-treat/

https://www.wildmedcenter.com/blog/skull-fractures

https://www.ems1.com/ems-training/articles/use-avpu-scale-to-determine-a-patients-level-of-consciousness-FVpjgzNGwSJAGoeQ/

https://www.brainline.org/article/managing-behavior-problems-during-brain-injury-rehabilitation

https://www.mayoclinic.org/healthy-lifestyle/fitness/expert-answers/heart-rate/faq-20057979

https://www.wildmedcenter.com/blog/traumatic-brain-injuries

https://www.backpacker.com/skills/the-cure-head-injuries

https://medcoer.com/concussions-are-sometimes-difficult-to-self-diagnose-leading-to-3-common-errors-that-can-cost-the-person-in-the-long-run/

https://www.mayoclinic.org/diseases-conditions/frostbite/symptoms-causes/syc-20372656

https://www.mayoclinic.org/diseases-conditions/frostbite/symptoms-causes/syc-20372656

https://www.healthline.com/health/frostnip#outlook

https://awls.org/wilderness-medicine-case-studies/frostbite-prevention-and-management

https://www.drugs.com/cg/frostbite-aftercare-instructions.html

https://blog.nols.edu/2015/08/11/preventing-and-treating-heat-illness

https://southeastwildernessmedicine.com/blog/heat-exhaustion-heat-stroke-concerned/

http://wildernessusa.com/learn/health-and-safety/heat-stroke/

https://www.britannica.com/story/can-you-drink-water-from-a-cactus

https://en.wikipedia.org/wiki/List_of_fatal_snake_bites_in_the_United_States#Snake_species

https://www.smithsonianmag.com/travel/american-safari-biggest-mammals-180958130/

https://www.cdc.gov/rabies/exposure/animals/index.html

https://americanhumane.org/fact-sheet/rabies-facts-prevention-tips

https://en.wikipedia.org/wiki/Category:Rodents_of_North_America

https://www.rentokil.com/au/rodent-borne-diseases/#plague

https://www.cdc.gov/plague/maps/index.html

https://www.rentokil.com/au/rodent-borne-diseases/#hantavirus

https://www.healthline.com/health/snake-bites

https://www.healthline.com/health/snake-bites#prevention

https://www.healthline.com/health/snake-bites#treatment

https://www.popularmechanics.com/adventure/outdoors/tips/a24203/eat-forage-food-wild-alone-history-channel/

https://www.foodpoisonjournal.com/food-poisoning-
watch/wilderness-underfoot-foodborne-illnesses-warm-
weather-heralds-the-start-of-food-poisoning-season/

https://share.upmc.com/2017/02/how-to-purify-water

https://medbroadcast.com/condition/getcondition/food-poisoning

https://www.redcross.org/content/dam/redcross/atg/PDFs/Take_a_
Class/WRFA_ERG_9781584806295.pdf

https://awls.org/injury-prevention/identifying-and-treating-poison-
ivy/

https://www.healthline.com/health/allergies/allergic-reaction-
treatment

https://www.redcross.org/take-a-class/cpr/performing-cpr/hands-
only-cpr

https://nhcps.com/lesson/cpr-first-aid-aed-choking-adults/

https://www.redcross.org/take-a-class/cpr/performing-cpr/cpr-steps

https://www.saintlukeskc.org/health-library/first-aid-rescue-
breathing

https://www.crisis-medicine.com/not-tourniquet-without-windlass/

https://sunrisehospital.com/about/newsroom/how-to-make-a-
tourniquet

https://cpraedcourse.com/course/cpr-certification/

https://www.wildmedcenter.com/blog/wmtc-evacuation-levels-
explained

FIRST AID

HANDBOOK

How to Heal from Urban Accidents

BRANDA NURT

Introduction

One Monday morning, a suburban woman named Jenny woke up feeling pretty refreshed. A little groggy and grumpy, but that's pretty much to be expected from waking up on a Monday morning. She put off her alarm, bathed, dressed up, and went out to face life, as we all do. She hurriedly ate her piece of toast and said goodbye to her dog without much fussiness. If she had known it would be the last goodbye she ever gave her beloved dog while alive, perhaps it would have been more dramatic. But I am getting ahead of myself.

Jenny rode the bus downtown to the city's commercial center. She had an important presentation and couldn't be late. During the bus trip, Jenny felt some discomfort in her chest area, which she dismissed as normal indigestion. It was not uncommon for Jenny to feel such discomfort, especially after rushing a meal. Still, this one seemed to be much more persistent, despite her swallowing and beating her chest repeatedly. But she ignored it, and after a while, it seemed to subside. Nerves, she reckoned. She did have an important presentation about business prospects in her market sector today, and she wasn't exactly on time yet.

Jenny finally got to her workplace, signed in to her cubicle, and gathered all necessary files for the presentation. All the while, the pain in her chest was periodically throbbing but she ignored it as just "stress."

She organized herself and her files just in time, as she was buzzed by her superior that it was time for the presentation. Jenny walked in confidently to the meeting room, full of 13 men and women, and plugged in her laptop. She was just about to begin her presentation when the pain in her chest flared and struck suddenly for the third time. This time it was no gentle throbbing; it was a powerful searing sensation radiating from her chest to her arms, her heart feeling like the hooves of a maniac horse were pounding it. Jenny collapsed onto the floor. As you'd expect, panic ensued. Freakish panic. This is not what you'd expect on your regular Monday. Confused silence. Chaos. Finally, someone got the idea to call Emergency Medical Services. The paramedics say they're on their way and to start her on first aid CPR if there is anyone conversant with first aid resuscitation. No one volunteers, because no one knows. A whole group of 13 bright minds and no one knows. In the excruciating minutes that follow, everyone watches Jenny on the floor, not moving, and there's absolutely nothing they could do. Not a single thing.

Finally, the paramedic arrives and starts simply doing "weird" things to her, including compressing her chest with their hands in weird motions and using shock thingy paddles. They rush her to the hospital at full speed, but it's too late. She doesn't make it. Jenny died en route to the hospital of her cardiac arrest. Jenny's demise is just one of the millions who die due to cardiac arrests. The paramedics shake his head, sighs, and says, "You know, if she had been given first aid, she just might have made it."

This book is designed to make you understand the power of first aid, its purpose, and its application in various forms. There are many ways to tell you why you must know first aid and reasons to read this book, but the simplest is this:

By the end of this book, if you're one of the thirteen partners witnessing Jenny's heart attack (who is fictional by the way), you would know what to do to save her. You would know how to handle that. And most importantly, you would save Jenny from an untimely death.

There is nothing nobler than that.

Chapter 1

First Aid: What is it all about?

First aid is defined as the emergency care that is at once given to an injured person. First aid is often given to individuals suffering from a medical emergency to mitigate injuries and prevent future disabilities. In various serious cases, first aid is what is necessary to keep the victim alive until the hospital is reached. First aid is simply the aid and basic medical care offered to anyone that is experiencing a sudden illness or injury. First aid even includes the support offered to someone experiencing a medical emergency until the medical team or paramedics arrive. Everyone must have at least a basic understanding of first aid. This is because it is virtually impossible to determine when an accident will take place. Accidents, by definition, are incidents that occur by chance, without deliberate intent that often leads to damage or injury. Accidents can happen at any place and at any time. It can happen in the workplace; it can happen at home; it can even happen in the middle of the street.

Many people believe there is nothing more to first aid than slapping a band-aid on a cut or calling the emergency line in cases of an incident. Some will say it is pouring water over a person's head while some people believe it is giving room to an injured person and not overcrowding him. It is why people who perform the basics of first aid, such as giving CPR, are considered heroes, not that they are not. First aid is a wide term that encompasses giving help and medical support to not just injured people but also those who are sick. First aid is more than a skill set. It also requires discretion and the ability to decide what the appropriate response to a certain situation or incident is.

But how long has first aid being in existence, and where did it originate from? We will discuss that in the next subheading.

History of First Aid

First aid was first introduced by St. John Ambulance in 1879 in the United Kingdom. Professor Esmarch gave five lectures in 1882, which were translated to English from German by the daughter of Queen Victoria, Princess Christian. Smith Elder and his partners eventually published the translated lectures with the title 'First Aid to the Injured.'

The First Aid Organization was first set up in Scotland in 1882 by St Andrew. The organization aimed to reduce the pains of the injured and the ill during times of war and peace. The organization also strove to take the needed steps necessary to take care of its patients. The rules and regulations put in place to manage the first aid organization were written by Sir George Beatson and released in 1891. In 1908, St. John and St. Andrew agreed to join forces, and together they worked and set up first aid care in several places in the United Kingdom and Scotland.

Esmarch, who was born in 1823, was the pioneer of civil first aid. He became a physician in 1848, furthered his studies and was appointed a specialist in the fields of ophthalmology and surgery in 1854. Esmarch was particularly interested in first aid and military surgery. Because he was an important emergency surgeon in the 19th century, he moved up the ranks to the surgeon-general of the German army during the French-German war. Also, a consulting surgeon in the military hospitals, he was well known in matters involving military surgery and hospital management. Doctor Mayor of Lausanne created the triangular bandage, but it became commonly used in the 1830s due to the approval of Esmarch. He was also, allegedly, the creator of the ice bag, thus bagging the nickname, the Ice Bag.

According to Esmarch, first aid aimed to protect the soldier's wounds from unsanitary elements as they were transported from the battlefield to the hospital. By covering the wound, Esmarch believed the soldier's injuries are protected from the sun, bugs, dust, and any other thing that can infect the wounds. His theory was that the move from the site of the accident to the place of care can greatly worsen the injuries.

When the First International Geneva Convention held in the mid-19th century, the Red Cross was formed. The Red Cross was created to help those who are sick and treat the fallen soldiers on the battlefield. Several soldiers were taught how to help their fellow soldiers before medical help arrived. The term first aid did not exist until about ten years after the First International Convention. In 1878, an army surgeon proposed that civilians be trained in 'premedical treatment.' The implementation of his idea brought, not just the term, but the deployment of civilian ambulances and personnel in Britain for the police, mines, and railways.

Now, several years later, the first aid skills have grown greatly. There is now very little difference between first aid practices and emergency medicine. Ambulances are now manned by personnel called paramedics or emergency medical technicians, EMTs, who have received advanced training.

Why You Should Learn First Aid

In several studies undertaken, it has been concluded that at least 8 out of every 10 parents out there admit too little to no knowledge of first aid procedures, which would undoubtedly save their children's lives in the event of an accident.

An article was recently published in the Irish Examiner on the 14th of May told the story of a grandfather saving a child with the knowledge and skills he got from first aid training. On his way to work, the man who has two grandchildren of his own, noticed a woman who was calling for help on an early Wednesday morning. The concerned man stopped and offered his assistance. The woman who had two children in her car was hardly able to get out the words explaining that one of the children is choking. The panic-stricken mother could not even open the doors. Armed with first aid knowledge Paul got the choking child out of the car and placed her over his knees. Hitting her shoulder blades sharply, he was able to remove the jelly sweet that was stuck in her throat. The distressed mother and child then found their way to the hospital for a checkup.

This instance is one of many that testifies to the importance of first aid. Imagine what would have happened to the three-year-old child if Paul had not stopped. What would have happened to the child if he had stopped but had no knowledge and no first aid training. Were the odds in the child's favor that they would have gotten to the hospital on time? Thanks to Paul's first aid training and refresher courses, they did not have to find out. In the words of the local hero, "that first aid move is one of the easiest techniques to learn, and you would be surprised how easily it sticks in your mind for when you need it. You don't think you will ever need to use it, but it is always in the back of your mind."

It is important that everyone have at least a basic understanding of first aid and how to implement it. The implementation of first aid practices saves lives every day. A very good example is the life that 19-year-old Megan James saved. Strolling with her son near Harbor Walk in Seaham, Megan heard a call for help. Wondering what was going on, she peeked around the corner and saw an unconscious man lying on the side of the road. The man's friend tried to help, but without proper first aid knowledge, he could not perform CPR properly. Confident in her skills because she took CPR classes when she had her child, Megan took over the CPR compressions, counting over and over like she had been taught. Finally, the man came about and took a deep breath. Just about then, the paramedics arrived and took the man to the hospital. They did inform Megan that her timely intervention saved the man's life.

Having even a rudimentary understanding of first aid is important because it helps to prevent the further deterioration of an injury before help arrives. Accidents happen anywhere and at any time. Take the experience of Richard Buff as an example. It all happened on a cool Saturday evening, the fourth of July, to be exact when Richard and his family were on their way home from a kid's birthday party in Monte Lake. Man, wife, and young sons were cruising on Highway 97 and found themselves behind three motorcycles. Wanting to overtake the car ahead of them, two of the bikers successfully passed the car ahead over the double solid pine that was near Duck Range Road. The third cyclist was not so lucky. In a tragic case of the wrong move at the wrong time, he peeked out and collided head-on with the grey oncoming car in his path. The resulting crash was loud enough to scare the pants off anyone, 'like a grenade going off,' it was described. Any other person would freak out or completely freeze in shock, but not Richard. Much unlike those 8 parents, Richard had recently completed his level three occupational first aid course and had even gotten a certification should any of his young sons ever need help. Pulling the car over immediately, Richard, the first aid hero, ran over to the car and checked on the young female driver. Confirming that she was not critically injured, he went over to the motorcyclist. The scene was quite a horrific one. One of the legs of the cyclist had been completely severed off right above the knees. While everyone stood around in shock at a complete loss of what to do, Richard called on his training and put to use skills he had learned but hoped he would never have to use. He got a belt from one of the bystanders and made a tourniquet on the severed leg. He handed that over to one of the two other bikers who had scaled through. He then checked the fallen biker for other life-threatening injuries. Just like he had been taught, Richard put the injured biker's elbows on the ground, raised his head, and slowly rolled him to a supine position to fully check him over. Thankfully, an off-duty nurse came over and could assist Richard in finding the severed leg and icing it immediately. The quick and informed actions of Richard, without a doubt, saved the biker's life. It possibly even saved the biker's leg. The knowledge of first aid is instrumental in ensuring that injuries that occur due to accidents do not deteriorate further, leading to loss of limbs or worse, of lives.

Like the incident above, the quick thinking and acquired skill set of Richard Buff ensured that the motorcyclist did not bleed to death on the highway. It ensured that when he arrived at the hospital, the doctors didn't waste precious minutes checking for vital signs and internal injuries when they could just start working on trying to save his legs. It even undoubtedly ensured that he did not die out there on the asphalt while everyone was busy trying to save his leg due to internal bleeding.

The Goal of First Aid

First aid is aimed at offering help towards sick or injured people. It is the immediate attention offered to a person immediately after an accident or an illness. The care given to a person between the time of an incident and the arrival of an ambulance can mean the difference between life and death and partial or full recovery.

The aims of first aid are simple. They are:

To Preserve Life

This is the most important principle of first-aid practices. It is why the first aid practices are established in the first place. The preservation of life requires the application of emergency practices to make sure that the victim is not in mortal danger, and the accident or incident is not fatal. The preservation of life also includes your life as first aid practices do not encourage that put your own life in danger while trying to save someone else's. The preservation of life encourages you to check and perform a quick assessment and check for dangers that might occur to yourself, the injured person, as well as bystanders, should the situation escalate. When in doubt, it is better to stand down and call for the assistance of a medical professional.

To Prevent the Worsening of Injuries

First aid works to prevent the worsening and further decline of the victim's injuries and health. It is important to keep the victim still to avoid aggravating their injury or from further complicating unseen injuries.

To Promote Recovery

There are various steps you can take as a first aider to reduce the recovery time of the patient and lessen lasting damage and scarring. A classic example is the quick application of cold water to a burn immediately to reduce the chances of scarring. It also helps speed up the healing process.

To Protect the Unconscious

These three aims are abbreviated and known as the three P's. While first aid has several limitations, it is what can save many people from death or serious permanent injury, all over the world in various medical emergencies.

Several medical cases deteriorate because bystanders, relatives, co-workers, passersby do not know what to do. They hesitate or are too timid to try, and that often leads to the needless deaths or chronic injuries of victims. Injured or sick people need assistance immediately. The quick action and quick thinking stand to make a difference in saving lives and limbs. Victims of accidents or injuries who are not breathing well or who are bleeding heavily require immediate assistance to increase their chances of a speedy recovery.

As first aid emergencies are often unexpected, it is important to remain calm and not panic. The quick action provided to the victim without a lot of delays is what is best for the victim. Careful and deliberate action, taken with thought and not as a reflex due to panic, goes a long way in helping the victim. The calm and collected actions of the first aider will also help reassure the bystanders that everything will be alright and reduce the general panic level and anxiety of the crowd.

Many times, people hesitate to offer help because they are afraid of being sued. Several governments, like that of Australia, are working on and enacting laws that protect the first aiders. There is still no successful litigation case against the first aider in Australia. The first aiders are protected as a 'Good Samaritan,' protected by the wrongs act 1958 (Victoria), the wrongs act 1936 (SA) of legislation, the civil liability Act of 2002 (NSW) to mention a few. This protection is effective with some conditions such as:

- It protects first aiders that deliver the care they are trained to deliver.

- It protects first aiders who work to the best of their ability and within reasonable limits.

- It protects first aiders who acted in good faith and in the best interest of the victim.

The Good Samaritan Laws

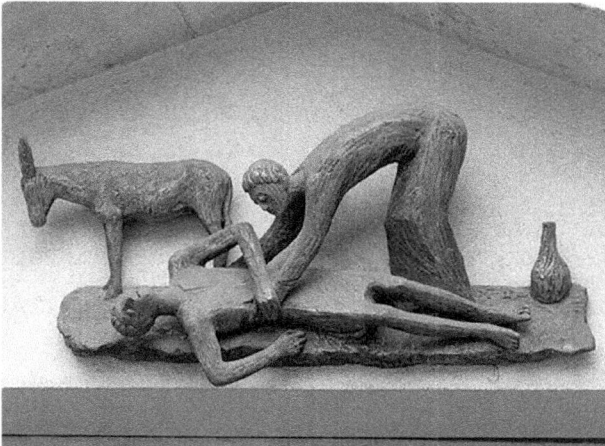

Several laws have been implanted to protect first aiders or those who assist victims of accidents and injuries within the limit. These laws are called 'The Good Samaritan' laws. The Good Samaritan laws aim to overcome bystander's reluctance to assist a victim in need because they might get sued or prosecuted for any unintentional injuries that result in the aid they rendered.

Several states and countries have implemented the Good Samaritan laws. In Canada, the Good Samaritan laws make sure that no form of persecution comes to the securer or first aider that helps a victim willingly. The presence and effectiveness of such laws encourage passersby to help those who are in need because they cannot be sued for any wrongdoing while caring for the victim.

Good Samaritan laws are available in almost every country. It varies in accordance with the legal principles already in place, such as parental rights, consent, and the right to refuse treatment. For the most part, the laws of Good Samaritan do not protect medical personnel, but it provides cover to professional rescuers who are working in a volunteer capacity.

Extracted from the Bible, the Good Samaritan name and law was coined from a parable told in Luke 10:29-37, which spoke about the help a man from Samaria offered a fellow traveler of different ethnic and religious background who had been robbed, beaten and left for dead by bandits. In the same vein, everyone is expected to render assistance to their neighbors irrespective of tribe, race, or any other affiliations in times of need. The Good Samaritan laws not only protect those who help the ill and the injured, but it also holds those who look the other way to the affliction of others responsible.

There is a great deal of similarity in the Good Samaritan laws of several countries. In spite of said similarities, there are also glaring differences. The Austrian Good Samaritan laws protect the rescuer only if the actions of the said rescuer is not influenced by hard drugs or alcohol. Not all states in Australia adhere to the same type of Good Samaritan laws.

While there are no recognized Good Samaritan laws in New South Wales, the efforts of good Samaritans are recognized in Victoria. They are protected so long as their actions were taken in good faith. In Belgium, not only does the Good Samaritan law protect first aiders from prosecution, but it also holds all its citizens to the task of helping their fellow man in need. However, that is only as long as they are not putting themselves or other people who are nearby in danger.

Canada provides leeway to all the provinces to create a Good Samaritan law that suits their province. Many provinces made use of the Good Samaritan Law of Ontario, Nova Scotia's Volunteer Services Act, British Columbia's, Alberta's Emergency Medical Aid Act, and so on. Despite several acts and laws to draw from, there are regions like Yukon and Nunavut that lack good and detailed Good Samaritan laws.

China originally had no Good Samaritan laws, but when several cases occurred, the government was forced to reconsider. One of such cases is the Peng Yu incident. The Peng Yu incident, which was a civil lawsuit, occurred in 2006 and found its way to the Nanjing District court in 2007.

The incident occurred on the 20th of November when Peng Yu helped Xu Shoulan, who fell while alighting from the bus. Like a gentleman, Peng Yu assisted Xu Shoulan to the hospital and contributed 200 RMB as part of the hospital payment. Xu Shoulan was diagnosed with a fractured femur and was duly informed that she needed a femur replacement surgery. She then demanded that Peng Yu reimburse her medical fees. When Peng Yu refused to meet her demands, she sued him for personal injury compensation accusing him of instigating her fall. The case was then presented to the court when several out of court mediation failed.

On the first of April 2007, the case was brought before the Gulou District Court in Nanjing. Xu declared before the court that she saw Peng knock into her. Fervently denying the allegation, Peng insisted that he only went to her after she had fallen. Chen Erchun, the eyewitness who was there at the scene, agreed with Peng, saying that Xu's fall was completely on her own without any collision. He further restated that he also helped them in getting in contact with Xu's relatives. Xu refuted Chen's statements, insisting that Peng had shoved her and caused her fall. Peng Yu finally admitted to accidentally knocking against Xu leading to the end of the court proceedings in March 2008. He then settled to pay 10,000 yuan as reimbursement to Xu Shoulan.

The public outcry condemned the actions of the court and its support of Xu Shoulan despite the lack of evidence against Peng. Even when he tried to help, he was still forced to pay for damages because the court believed that 'no one in good conscience would help someone else unless they felt guilty about something.' The decision of the court revealed to the Chinese citizens how they are setting themselves up for legal trouble if they tried to help a person in need and said person sues them for damages. The decision of the court that year had a devastating effect three years later when it caused the death of a two-year-old child.

On a cloudy October afternoon, Wang Yue wandered away from her home in Foshan while her mother hurriedly collected her laundry during a thunderstorm. Several closed-circuit television cameras caught the little girl as she wandered into the busy market street. A few moments after she appeared on the screen, she was knocked to the ground by a white van. The van driver paused for a moment but did not get out of the van. Instead, he slowly pulled forward and ran over Wang with his rear wheels. Soon after, another large truck ran over Wang's legs with both its front and back tires. At that time, 18 people passed by Wang, but while some paused and stared, none stopped to help her until a rubbish scavenger Chen Xianmei came along. Wang was sent to the hospital for treatment but eventually succumbed to her wounds and died eight days later. When the video was released, there was a huge outcry towards the moral decline of society, the callousness of the 18 people who passed the girl by, doing nothing to help. During a survey that circulated at that time, 88% of the people polled believed that Wang died due to the growing indifference of people towards one another in China.

In comparison, 71% of them believed those passersby were probably afraid of getting into trouble themselves, citing the high-profile PengYu incident as a classic example. This led to several talks within the government, which would not only protect those who tied to help from lawsuits but also punish those who could help but failed to in situations such as Wang's. China's national Good Samaritan law became effective as Clause 184 in Civil Law General Principles on the 1st of October 2017.

The Good Samaritan Laws in Finland, the Finland Rescue Act, states that a duty to rescue is a general duty to act and assist in rescue activities to the best of one's abilities. Included within the Act is a principle of proportionality that demands that professionals offer immediate help even more than the layperson. It is a crime punishable under the law in Germany to ignore a person in need. German laws also stipulate that the help provided cannot and will not be sued even in cases where it made the situation worse or did not check all the first aid criteria. In an attempt to further encourage people to help their fellow neighbor in need, first aiders are covered under the German Statutory Accident Insurance should they suffer any injury or loss or damages.

Of the 480,000 road accidents that occurred in India in 2016, 150,000 of them were fatal, leading to the loss of lives. The Good Samaritan laws provide legal cover to the citizens of Karnataka to assist accident victims with the emergency medical care needed within the 'Golden Hour.' It also encourages people to act even if they are not successful.

Other countries that have enacted the Good Samaritan Law in one form or another include:

- Ireland which protects the first aiders without demanding a duty to intervene

- Israel which obliges its citizens to help a person in danger or call for help at the very least while protecting the people who acted in good faith

- Romania who passed the bill in 2006 stating that anyone who is without medical training which offers first aid voluntarily on the instructions of medical personnel or own knowledge is not subject to penal or civil lawsuits

- The United States whose Good Samaritan Laws vary from state to state

- The United Kingdom whose common laws provide legal cover for first aiders. While the courts of the United Kingdom are reluctant to take action against those who stepped forward and offered to help in situations that require medical attention, it has no problem punishing those who stood by and did nothing, especially when a situation rapidly deteriorated right in front of them.

As you can see, First Aid is not only a useful and literally life-saving skill to learn; it is also a legally protected act as well. Not only are you saving a life, but you are also insured from legal repercussions whatsoever. One thing you must, however, the note is that you MUST not perform first Aid steps if a patient actively REFUSES your help. This might be due to a variety of reasons, but it is within the victim's right to refuse treatment. Consent is of paramount importance, especially for conscious patients.

Now that you are acquainted with the aim, scope, history, and legalities of First Aid, it is time to talk about the type of conditions and injuries. First Aid treatments can be useful. All of this will be discussed in the next chapter.

Chapter 2

Health Issues: Injuries and Medical Conditions that Require First Aid

A s stated earlier above, first aid is the first line of emergency health care given to an injured person or sick person. Hence, an understanding of the different types of injuries there are, their causes and symptoms are absolutely necessary to identify what nature of illness you're dealing with and how to treat it successfully. In this chapter, we're going to be looking at the most likely types of injuries and conditions you're going to come across, and how to prevent them in some cases, to further aid first aid treatments.

Cardiovascular Diseases

Cardiovascular diseases or CVD is a general term that encompasses the various conditions that affect the heart and blood vessels. It is often associated with the buildup of fatty deposits within the arteries, which leads to atherosclerosis, among others. Cardiovascular diseases can also be linked to damage caused to the arteries in major organs of the body such as the brain, heart, kidneys, and the eyes. Even though cardiovascular disease is one of the leading causes of death in the United Kingdom, it can be largely prevented by leading a healthy lifestyle. Even more than the United Kingdom, cardiovascular diseases are the number one cause of death globally as many people die from CVDs than they do from any other cause. In 2016, an estimated 17.9 million people died from several cardiovascular diseases, thus representing 31% of all the global deaths. Of those 17.9 million, 85% of them were as a result of heart attacks. As you can see, heart attacks are a major medical condition you should know about.

The Heart

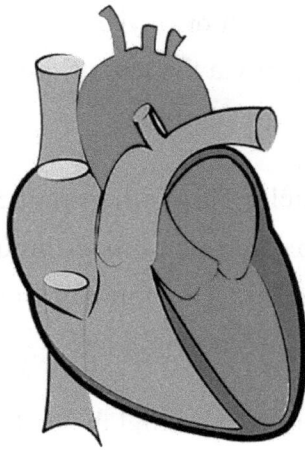

The heart is one of the major organs of the body. It is a muscular organ that is just about the size of your fist. It is located just behind the breastbone, slightly to the left between the lungs. It is a very important organ protected by the ribs, the breastbone, and the spine. The heart beats at about 70 times a minute and more than three billion times a lifetime, pumping blood through a network of arteries and veins. They all comprise of the cardiovascular system. The heart is divided into two parts and four chambers:

The Right Atrium: Obtaining blood from the veins is the right atrium. The blood collected is then propelled to the right ventricle.

The Right Ventricle: The blood which leaves the right atrium goes into the right ventricle. It is from the right ventricle that blood moves to the lungs in order to obtain oxygen.

The Left Atrium: The blood in the lungs receives oxygen and becomes oxygen-rich or oxygenated. The oxygenated blood returns to the heart via the left atrium. The left atrium passes the blood to the left ventricle.

The Left Ventricle: This is the strongest part of the heart. It dispenses the oxygen-rich blood throughout the body via a number of arteries. The forceful contractions of the left ventricle make the blood pressure.

As the blood makes it rounds around the body, it finds its way back to your heart through the veins, and the cycle continues. That cycle is a process known as circulation.

Running along the muscles of the heart are the coronary arteries. The coronary arteries are the arteries that supply the heart of its own blood. There is also a web of nerve tissue surrounding the heart that conducts a series of complex signals which control the contraction and relaxation of the heart.

Types of Cardiovascular Diseases

Cardiovascular diseases are a group of disorders of not just the heart but also the blood vessels. They include::

- Coronary heart disease

- Cerebrovascular diseases, also known as a stroke or a transient ischemic attack

- Peripheral arterial disease

- Aortic disease

The shared behavioral risk factors that the listed cardiovascular diseases have in common include physical laziness, an unwholesome diet, tobacco use, and the extreme intake of alcohol. The results of these behavioral lifestyles show in elevated blood glucose levels, obesity, overweight, and raised blood lipids.

1. Coronary Heart Disease

Coronary heart diseases are diseases that occur due to the obstruction of blood rich in oxygen to the heart muscle. The blood flow might be blocked or reduced. This increases the workload of the heart, and the heart ends up strained.

When the blood supply of the heart is blocked or disturbed because of the buildup of fatty substances in the arteries, coronary heart disease occurs. The constant presence of fatty substances in meals leads to an increased amount of fatty substances that are placed in the arteries. As time passes, the arterial walls become padded with fatty deposits. The fatty deposits are known as atheroma, and the padding up of the arteries is through a continuous process known as atherosclerosis.

Several lifestyle factors can lead to atherosclerosis like smoking and the regular intake of a disproportionate amount of alcohol. Several underlying conditions, like high cholesterol, high blood pressure, otherwise known as hypertension and diabetes, also increase the chances of an individual getting atherosclerosis.

The severely reduced blood flow can lead to chest pains or angina, which is caused by the restricted blood flow to the heart muscle. When the arteries of the heart are completely blocked due to a blood clot, a heart attack happens. Stress or overexertion of an individual with narrowed coronary arteries can lead to what is known as stable angina pectoris. The blockages to the heart prevent the heart from receiving the extra oxygen it needs for the strenuous activity the body is currently undergoing. The chest pains usually dissipate with rest. When the chest pain or discomfort is new or worsening or occurring even at rest, it is usually indicative of unstable angina pectoris. It is an emergency situation that is often indicative of a heart attack, cardiac arrest, or serious abnormal heart rhythm.

2. Strokes And TIAs

A stroke occurs when the blood supply to a part of the brain is cut off. It is a serious and life-threatening condition that can lead to brain damage and even death. A TIA is a transient ischemic attack or a mini-stroke. It is similar to a stroke, but the blood flow is only disrupted and not cut off. When the blood supply to the brain is disrupted, restricted, or stopped, the brain cells in that particular region begins to die. This can lead to brain injury, disability, and even death. There are two main causes for strokes

Ischemic: This occurs when the blood supply to the brain is interrupted due to a blood clot. It accounts for a large portion, about 85% of all stroke cases.

Hemorrhagic: This is a stroke that occurs when the blood vessel which supplies the brain bursts.

The major difference between a TIA and a stroke is that a TIA does not last as long, its effects often lasting from a few minutes to a few hours. It is often fully resolved within 24 hours. A TIA is often a warning sign that a full stroke is not far behind in the nearest future. A TIA occurs when one of the blood vessels that carry oxygen-rich blood to the brain is blocked. The blockage is often a result of a blood clot that is formed elsewhere in the body and travels to the blood vessels that supply the brain. The blockage may also be as a result of pieces of fatty materials or air bubbles. There are certain factor that increases the chances of having a TIA which include:

- smoking

- high blood pressure or hypertension,

- obesity,

- high cholesterol levels,

- diabetes,

- regular drinking of an excessive amount of alcohol

- atrial fibrillation, a type of irregular heartbeat

People who are over the age of 55 years as well as those with Asian, African, and Caribbean descent, are at higher risk of having a TIA.

3. Peripheral Arterial Disease

Peripheral arterial disease or PAD is one that occurs due to a blockage of the arteries to the limbs, often to the legs. It occurs due to the build-up of deposits of fat in the arteries. This then restricts the blood supply to the legs. It is also known as a peripheral vascular disease (PVD). It rarely presents with symptoms, but some report a painful ache in their legs when walking. Said pain disappears after a couple of minutes' rest. That is called 'intermittent claudication' in medical terms. The pain ranges from mild to severe and usually disappears when the legs are rested for a couple of minutes. While both legs can be affected at the same time, the pain is usually more severe in one leg. The other symptoms that PAD presents are:

- loss of hair on the hands and feet

- weakness and numbness in the legs

- slow-growing and brittle toenails

- open sores or ulcers on the feet and legs that do not heal

- shiny skin

- changing the skin color on the legs to pale or blue

- erectile dysfunction in men

- the shrinking of the leg muscles (muscle wasting)

A peripheral arterial disease is a form of cardiovascular disease due to its effect on the blood vessels. The large deposits of fatty droplets in the walls of the leg arteries lead to a blockage of the arteries. The fatty deposits are then made up of cholesterol and other waste substances. Some factors that increase the chances of PAD include:

- Smoking as the most significant risk factor

- Type 1 and type 2 diabetes

- High blood pressure

- High cholesterol

- Old age

4. Aortic Disease

There is a group of diseases that afflict the aorta. They are called aortic diseases. The aorta is not only the largest blood vessel of the body, running from the chest to the tummy; it is also one of the most important. The aorta transports blood all over the body from the heart. There are several types of aortic diseases, but aortic aneurysm is the most common. The weakness and outward swelling of the aorta is the most common characteristic of an aortic aneurysm. The most dangerous aortic aneurysm is the abdominal aortic aneurysm. Early detection is the only prevention against the potentially fatal disease.

Abdominal aortic aneurysm swells and can burst anytime, leading to severe bleeding.

While it is not yet fully clear why an abdominal aortic aneurysm happens, certain factors increase its risk. Men over the age of 66 and women over 70 with any of the risk factors listed below are at risk of an abdominal aortic aneurysm.

- Chronic obstructive pulmonary disease

- High blood pressure

- High blood cholesterol

- Family history of abdominal aortic aneurysm

- A history of stroke

- Cardiovascular disease

- If they smoke or have previously smoked.

- Abdominal aortic aneurysm does not often present with obvious symptoms, but some people with AAA have complained of the following

- A heartbeat-like feeling in the stomach

- Persistent stomach pain

- Constant pain in the lower back

- A ruptured abdominal aortic aneurysm can cause

- A serious ache in the tummy and throb in the lower back.

- Dizziness

- A rather rapid heartbeat

- Pale, sweaty and clammy skin

- Passing out or fainting

- Wheezing breath

Breathing Emergencies

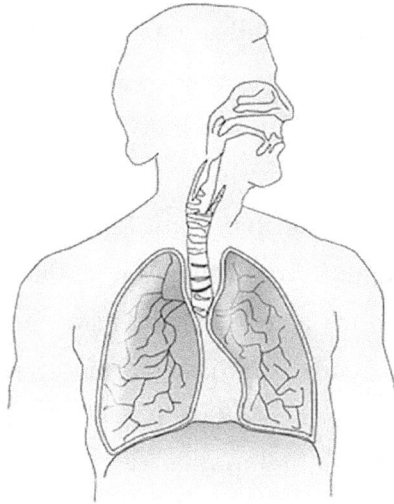

The body requires a continuous supply of oxygen to function. Oxygen enters the body through breathing, which is the process of inhaling oxygen and exhaling carbon dioxide. The oxygen inhaled mixes with and is transferred into the blood. The blood then carries the oxygen throughout the body to various parts of the body. Without oxygen, all parts of the body would shut down and stop working, leading to the untimely death of the victim. This is why breathing is very important. Everyone breathes through the nose and the mouth. The air then travels down through the throat, down the windpipe, and into the lungs. The pathway from the nose and mouth to the lungs is called the airway. The airway is important, and any blockage must be immediately removed, or it might cause severe damage to the victim. That is why it is important to make sure that regardless of age, air must reach the lungs whenever breathing emergencies occur.

Breathing emergencies occur whenever a person cannot easily pass air into the lungs. Some breathing emergencies greatly reduce the access of air into the lungs while some cut off the access to oxygen in the lungs completely. The result of little to no air in the lungs means the heart stops beating, and blood does not flow to the body. Without oxygen to the brain, the brain cells die within four to six minutes. Lack of oxygen to the brain longer than that can lead to permanent brain damage or death. While the majority of adults experience a heart attack and their hearts stop beating, children and infants have healthy hearts, so it is important to recognize breathing difficulties in children because that is the stoppage of the heart is usually as a result of breathing problems.

Difficulties breathing is often one of the first signals indicative of a bigger problem like a heart attack. Understanding the signals and having the necessary knowledge to provide care is usually key to preventing more serious problems. A conscious injured, or ill person will be able to answer your questions and indicate to you what the problem is. It becomes tricky if you are not able to communicate with the victim. This is why it is important to know the signals for breathing emergencies and know when to call for help.

Types Of Breathing Emergencies

There are two types of breathing emergencies:

Respiratory Distress: This is a condition whereby breathing is difficult.

Respiratory Arrest: This is a condition in which breathing stops.

Both respiratory distress and respiratory arrest are a type of breathing disorder. Respiratory distress is the most common type of breathing emergency. Respiratory distress can lead to respiratory arrest.

We all breathe normally without effort or thought to it. Unless under strenuous activity, breathing is usually regular without working too hard to catch a breath and a struggle to breathe. Children and infants breathe faster than adults as they have faster than normal breathing rates. A change in breathing pattern is also normal for infants as they have periodic breathing. Periodic breathing is a type of breathing where an infant's breathing pauses for as long as 10 seconds at a time. The pauses may be close together and are followed by a succession of shallow and rapid breaths. This type of breathing is quite common in premature babies in the first few weeks of life. Healthy full-term babes are not also strangers to periodic breathing. Periodic breathing happens mostly when the infant is deeply asleep. They may also happen when during light sleep or when the baby is awake. Breathing resumes normally for a baby with periodic breathing without prompting or intervention, and it goes away as the baby grows older. It is important to note that periodic breathing is not the same as apnea, where the breathing stops for at least 20 seconds. Breathing emergencies are usually identified by watching and listening to the person's breathing.

Causes of Respiratory Distress and Respiratory Arrest

Several factors can lead to respiratory distress and respiratory arrest. Some of those factors include:

- Choking due to a partially or completely obstructed airway

- Illness

- Several chronic conditions which can be long-lasting or frequently reoccurring

- Electrocution

- Irregular heartbeat

- Heart attack

- Injury to the head or the brain stem, lungs, chest or abdomen

- Allergic reactions

- Drug or alcohol overdose

- Poisoning

- Emotional distress

- Drowning

Chronic Obstructive Pulmonary Disease

The collection of chronic inflammatory diseases is known as chronic obstructive pulmonary diseases, otherwise known as COPD. COPD occurs when the airways to the lungs deteriorate and leads to the partial blockage of the airways. The dilapidation of the air sacs leads to their inability to fill with air as they should. This leads to difficulty breathing. COPD currently has no cure, but the effects can be managed with the proper medication. Signs of COPD include constant coughing, the production of sputum, wheezing, and trouble breathing.

Emphysema and chronic bronchitis are the two common COPD conditions. They usually go hand in hand and vary in severity.

The smoking of cigarettes has been proven to be the leading cause of chronic obstructive pulmonary disease. Other factors that may lead to chronic obstructive pulmonary disease are inhaling any kind of lung irritants, dust, chemicals, or pollution for a stretch of time. Anyone who has been identified with COPD also runs the risk of developing lung cancer, heart disease, and several other conditions.

The symptoms of COPD include:

- Coughing up a large amounts of mucus

- The tendency to get tired easily

- Poor appetite

- wheezing

- Shortness of breath

- Puckered lips for easier breathing as well as elevated shoulders and a crooked posture

- A rapid pulse

- Unintended weight loss in the later stages

- A rotund chest that is shaped like a barrel

- Confusion as a result of poor oxygen delivery to the brain.

- Swelling around the feet, ankles or the legs

Emphysema

Emphysema is a common type of COPD. It occurs due to the eradication of the alveoli and bronchioles at the smallest air passages of the airways due to prolonged exposure to the smoke of cigarettes, irritating gases, and particulate matter. This leads to the destruction of the air sacs. Various symptoms are indicative of emphysema, and they include trouble exhaling as well as shortness of breath. More severe cases manifest by restlessness, bewilderment or confusion, general body weakness, sudden cardiac arrest, to mention a few.

Chronic Bronchitis

Bronchitis occurs as a result of swollen air passages. It can be an acute or chronic condition. Chronic bronchitis is classified as a type of COPD and is determined when the victim constantly coughs with mucus for at least three months.

It is important to remember that acute bronchitis is not a type of COPD as it develops after a person has had a viral respiratory infection. It first distresses the nose, then the sinuses and the throat before it spreads to the lungs. Infants, children, the elderly, smokers, and individuals who are suffering from heart or lung diseases are most susceptible to acute bronchitis.

Symptoms of both the acute and the chronic bronchitis include

- Cough with mucus

- Chest discomfort

- Low fever

- Fatigue

- Worsening shortness of breath upon the activity

- Wheezing

- Symptoms for chronic bronchitis include

- Swelling in the ankle, the feet, and the leg

- Blue lips

- Constant respiratory infections like the colds and the flu.

Hyperventilation

Hyperventilation is easily recognized by the faster and shallower breathing of the victim. The hyperventilating victim is not getting enough oxygen to supply the body. When the body is lacking in oxygen, the victim begins to hyperventilate. This leads to a reduction in the carbon dioxide in the body and causes a change in the acidity of the blood.

Hyperventilating victims believe they are not breathing well or greeting enough air. This causes them to feel fear, anxiety, or confusion. They also complain of lightheadedness and a tingly feeling in their extremities, such as their toes and fingers. Hyperventilation often occurs due to an emotional upheaval such as fear, anxiety, or worry. Apart from emotional reactions, it can also occur as a result of severe bleeding that leads to the lack of oxygen, head injuries, or other forms of injuries like a high fever, lung or heart diseases, and diabetic emergencies. Hyperventilation can also be triggered due to strenuous exercises or an asthma attack.

Croup

Croup is a harsh and repetitive cough that affects children under the age of 5. It leads to the constriction of the airways and limits the passage of air. This then causes the child to emit an unusually sounding cough that ranges from a barking cough to a high-pitched wheeze. Croup is often an evening and nighttime illness.

Most of the time, croups are taken care of at home, and it usually dissipates by the use of cool air or mist treatment. In other cases, however, croup progresses very quickly from respiratory distress to respiratory arrest.

Epiglottitis

Epiglottis is even less common an infection than the croup that causes the swelling of the epiglottis. The epiglottis is found at the back of the tongue like a piece of cartilage that, when swollen, can block the windpipe and cause severe breathing problems. The bacteria Hemophilus influenzae causes an infection that leads to epiglottitis. Its symptoms are similar to that of croups, but it is a much more serious illness as it can result in death if the airway is completely blocked. Epiglottitis used to be a common disease for children between the ages of 2 to 6. The number of children infected in the United States had reduced drastically since the 1980s when the vaccines for H. influenzae type B became commonplace.

Epiglottitis often begins with a sore throat and a high fever in both children and adults. In order to breathe, anyone suffering from epiglottitis needs to sit up and lean forward with the chin thrust out. Other symptoms of epiglottitis include drooling, voice changes, difficulty swallowing, shaking, chills, and fever.

Environmental Emergencies

Disaster may strike at any time, and it is not always about diseases, illnesses, or injury. A great deal of our environment is relatively harmless. A weekend communing with nature can help you better appreciate the world we live in and the joys of nature, the clear blue skies, the crisp, cold air, the sun in your face, the sight of the mountains, the roar of the river, the flight of the animals and insects. They are all beautiful and relatively harmless, but that very beautiful, calm, and serene environment also carries disease-carrying insects as well as other biting creatures. Even though environmental emergencies can be avoided, accidents do occur.

The crisp air can lead to a cold-related injury, and the sun can cause a heat-related injury. Exposure to either side of the spectrum, both hot and cold, can cause a person to become seriously ill. Some factors can lead to either of them happening like physical activity, wind, humidity, clothing, working and living conditions, age as well as state of mind.

Once the symptoms of a cold-related or heat-related emergency appear, the situation deteriorates rapidly and can easily lead to death. Those who are at risk of heat-related or cold-related illnesses are those who work outside, those who are outdoorsy exercisers, the elderly, young children, and individuals with health problems. Those include conditions that lead to poor blood circulation and those who take medications that cause the elimination of water from the body (diuretics).

People often leave extreme hot or cold environments before they get ill, but some do not or cannot. Athletes and those who work outdoors keep on working and remain in those places even when they begin to feel ill. Those who live in buildings with poor ventilation, poor insulation, and poor heating and/or cooling systems are also highly susceptible to experiencing heat-related emergencies and cold-related illnesses. Many times, they may not even know that they are in danger of becoming sick.

Heat-Related Illnesses

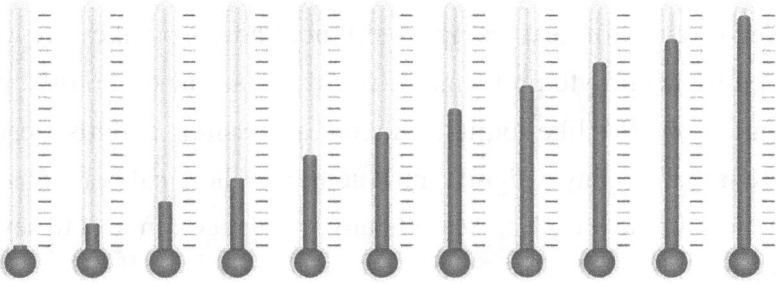

Overexposure to heat can lead to several illnesses such as heat cramps, heat exhaustion, heatstroke. These illnesses, in turn, lead to a loss of fluids and electrolytes, which upset the balance of the body and leads to the body breaking down.

Heat Cramps

Of all the heat-related illnesses, heat cramps are the least concerning. It is usually the body's first sign that the temperature is on the high side. Heat cramps are painful. They are the involuntary movement of the muscles causing involuntary muscle spasm. The spasms might be more intense and much more prolonged than typical nighttime leg cramps. The loss of fluids and electrolytes, no doubt, contributes to heat cramps. The muscles re most often affected are the calves, the arms, those of the abdominal wall, and the muscles in the back. During exercise, heat cramps might involve just about any muscle group.

The likelihood of heat cramps happening increase when working in a hot environment, especially activities that one is not used to doing. Another risk factor is the poor intake of salt while simultaneously sweating a great deal.

The exact cause of heat cramps is still not known, but they are likely related to electrolyte problems. Electrolytes are made up of several essential minerals like sodium, calcium, potassium, and magnesium. These minerals play a significant role in the chemical reactions that take place in the muscles. As such, any imbalance can lead to several problems.

The sweat that pours out of the body through the pores contains a great deal of sodium, and the intake of fluids without an adequate amount of sodium can lead to a severe low-sodium condition called hyponatremia.

Several symptoms can identify heat cramps. The muscle spasms that occur are usually:

- Painful

- Brief

- Involuntary

- Intermittent

- Often self-limited

Heat Exhaustion

Heat exhaustion is a more severe condition than heat cramps. It is a common problem for firefighters, athletes, factory works, and construction workers. It is also a concern for those who wear heavy clothing in a hot and humid environment. It occurs as a result of the loss of water and salt from the body, through exposure to high temperatures in combination with high humidity and strenuous physical activity. All of these cause the body to overheat and induces heavy sweating and a rapid pulse.

The heat that the body produces, combined with the heat of the environment, is what results in what is known as the body's core temperature. The body's core temperature is the body's internal temperature. The body is very good at regulating itself to match the environmental temperatures such as heat gain or heat loss as appropriate.

Whenever the weather is hot, the body can maintain its core temperature and cool itself majorly by sweating. When the sweat evaporates from the body, the body cools down, and the body temperature is regulated. However, in times of rigorous exercise or strenuous work in a hot and humid environment, the body is unable to cool itself effectively. In response, the mildest of heat-related illnesses, heat cramps occur. Heat cramps then progress and lead to heat exhaustion. If care is not given as soon as possible, heatstroke, the deadliest of the trio, soon comes next.

The signs and symptoms of heat exhaustion can suddenly develop or take its time, especially after a long exercise period. The signs and symptoms of heat exhaustion include

Humid and clammy skin with goosebumps even while in the not weather.

- Wooziness

- Heavy perspiration

- Fainting

- Fatigue

- Low blood pressure while standing

- A weak and rapid pulse

- Nausea

- Muscle cramps

- Headaches

Heatstroke

Heatstroke is the least common of heat-related illnesses. It is also the most severe of the three. When the signs of heat exhaustion are ignored, heat stroke happens. It often occurs during the summer and in warm climates when the body is severely overheated, and the core temperature is as high as 40C or 104F. Although uncommon, heat strokes require immediate attention because it can lead to severe damage to the heart, kidneys, muscles, and even the brain if ignored. Delay in treatment can lead to further deterioration and can even lead to the death of the victim.

- The signs and symptoms of heatstroke include

- Really elevated body temperature

- There is a sudden change in behavior and mental alertness of the victim. The victim begins to experience confusion, agitation, or slurred speech.

- The victim might even be delirious or experience seizures.

- Instead of hot and dry skin, there is a change in the sweating pattern of the victim, which leads to slightly moist skin.

- Nausea and vomiting

- Rapid breathing

- Flushed skin

- Headaches

- Increased heart rate.

Cold-Related Emergencies

The evolutionary process did not equip man to adapt to cold climates. Humans are more suited for warm climates. This is evident in the way our generally flat and angular shaped bodies, along with our long limbs, are designed to encourage heat loss. Humans are relatively hairless, which makes us able to lose heat easily. Transversely, this also makes us unable to handle the cold climate without proper clothing and a source of heat. This causes the body to malfunction, and it can lead to death. Cold related emergencies are not often recognized or treated immediately because the victims believe they can 'tough it out.'

The two types of cold-related emergencies are frostbite and hypothermia.

Frostbite

Exposure to extreme cold leads to frostbite. When any part of the body is left unprotected or bare to the chilly air, the body part begins to freeze. The gravity of frostbites depends on how long the body part has been exposed to the icy chill. It can lead to the loss of hands, fingers, arms, feet, toes as well as legs. Cold temperature lead to injuries in the skin as well as the underlying tissues. The parts of the body that are often left bare and uncovered, such as the toes, nose, cheeks, ears, fingers, chin, and so on, are often victims of frostbite. Even with gloves, the fingers are sometimes casualties of frostbite.

Frostbite can occur in various stages.

> **Frostnip**: Frostnip is the mildest form of frostbite. Prolonged exposure to cold can lead to numbness in the affected areas. Pain and tingling are experienced as the skin warms. Frostnip leaves no permanent damage to the skin.

Superficial frostbite: The superficial frostbite appears to be reddened skin, which turns white or pale. The skin begins to feel warm. That shows that there is serious skin involvement. Rewarming at this stage can cause mottled skin. It is also accompanied by stinging, burning, and swelling. After rewarming the skin, a fluid-filled blister may appear some 12-36 hours later.

Deep or severe frostbite: Deep frostbite occurs when the body is subjected to cold temperatures for long enough to cause all skin layers and the tissues beneath to become affected. This leads to the whitening or blush-grey color of the skin. Numbness, loss of awareness of pain, cold, or discomfort in the distressed areas are to be expected. The joints and muscles may also become frozen. After rewarming the distressed areas for 24 to 48 hours, large blisters may form. If that happens, the affected area will turn black and hard because the underlying tissues are dying.

Frostbite is a milder kind of cold injury, and it hardly ever causes permanent damage to the skin. The symptom of frostbite include:

- Cold skin and a prickling feeling at first

- Numbness

- Hard or waxy-looking skin

- Red, white or bluish-white skin

- Clumsiness due to muscle or joint stiffness

- In severe cases, blistering occurs after rewarming.

Hypothermia

Hypothermia does not require cold and frigid temperatures like frostbite before it affects a person. Hypothermia occurs as a result of the body's inability to maintain its core temperature. A wet body or a windy day are two common conditions that often lead to hypothermia. Without proper care, persons suffering from hypothermia will die. When the body is unable to generate heat fast and adequate enough to combat the environmental cool, hypothermia occurs. This causes the body to drop to very low temperatures. The normal body temperature is 37 degrees Celsius or 98.6°F, but when hypothermia sets in, the body temperature reduces drastically to 35 degrees Celsius or 95°F. The homeless, the sick, young children, and the elderly who reside in poorly heated homes are at most risk of suffering from hypothermia.

A drop in the body temperature leads to a malfunction of the major organs of the body. That includes the heart, the brain, the lungs, and in some cases the entire nervous system. A victim suffering from hypothermia does not become immediately aware of the condition. The confused thinking that is also related to hypothermia hinders self-awareness. The first sign of hypothermia is shivering. Shivering will occur almost immediately. The temperature of the body drops as the body's automatic defense against the cold, which is to warm itself, kicks in.

The symptoms of hypothermia include:

- Shivering

- Slow and shallow breathing

- A weak pulse

- Mumbling or slurred speech

- Drowsiness and very low energy

- Lack of coordination

- Loss of consciousness in severe cases

- Bright red, color skin.

Brain Injuries

Accidents occur all the time that may lead to an injury in the brain or spinal cord. A bat may swing at the wrong time; a punch might land in the wrong place; a foot might find its way to the head during a fight. Even apart from confrontations, there are environmental causes that can lead to brain injuries such as falling or tripping. Many victims of brain and spinal injuries might even dust themselves up and move on, without knowing they have been severely injured somewhere.

The brain and the spinal cord are what make up the central nervous system. The central nervous system is the power hub of the body. It is responsible for sending signals down to the rest of the body, receiving information from the sensory organs, processing the information received, and making the appropriate decision. The importance of the brain and spinal cord cannot be overemphasized. Any altercation to them, no matter how minute, can lead to great and many rimes irreversible changes to the individual.

The major parts of the brain are the cerebrum, the cerebellum, and the brainstem. The largest part of the brain is the cerebrum and it sits on top of all the other structures. It is one of the most important parts of the brain because it is the center for learning, language, sensory processing, and memory. The decision to raise your hand or swing your legs or make a voluntary movement is initiated in the cerebrum. The decision is then finetuned in the cerebellum. Located just below the hind part of the cerebrum is the cerebellum. The cerebellum not only coordinates movements and motor learning, but there is also evidence that shows that the cerebellum is involved in other non-motor functions. The brainstem, which is located in the lower part of the brain, goes on to form the spinal cord. The two major functions of the brainstem are to regulate heart rate and respiratory rate.

The functions of the brain are still a mystery to scientists as not everything about the brain is known. From the little that is known, it confirms that any damage to the brain is dangerous, but that to the brainstem is particularly life-threatening.

There are protective layers all around the brain called meninges. The meninges are tri-layered and are divided into the outermost layer, otherwise known as the fur a mater, the middle layer of the arachnoid, and the outermost layer or the pia mater. Between the arachnoid and the pia mater is the subarachnoid space. The subarachnoid space is full of the cerebrospinal fluid, CSF, which saves the brain from itself by ensuring it does not crush itself from its own weight. The CSF offers nutrients and removes waste.

The human skull consists of 22 bones, 14 of which make up the facial skeleton, and 8 make up the neurocranium of the braincase as it is otherwise known. The top and side neurocranium bones are the strongest, working hand in hand to protect the brain, the cerebrum, and the cerebellum especially, against damages. The brainstem exits the neurocranium into the vertebral column.

33 vertebrae make up the spine or the vertebral column, which runs from the base of the skull to the pelvis. The vertebrae are designed to not only support the body but also protect the spinal cord. The spinal cord, which is an extension from the brain stem, through the spinal canal, and into the vertebral column, is made up of nervous tissue. The spinal canal is filled with cerebrospinal fluid, CSF, which serves the same function in the spine as it does in the brain.

Head Injuries

Injuries to the brain and the spinal cord are usually caused by trauma to the head and the neck. Injuries to the scalp, face, and skull might be indications that there is an injury to the central nervous system, but that is not always the case. On the other side, there might be injuries to the central nervous system that are present even in the absence of head trauma. In cases of a fall or an accident, it is safer than the victims to be monitored closely for any head injury.

Fractures

Not all skull fractures are life-threatening but some are deceptive, seemingly normal but potentially fatal. Fractures are either open or closed. Open fractures expose the fractured bone to the environment by either tearing through the skin or through a laceration directly on the fracture. Any other type of fracture are closed fractures.

Not just as open and closed fractures, skull fractures can also be classified based on location and the number of the fracture. A linear fracture runs in a fairly straight line without bone displacement. A depressed fracture, on the other hand, displaces the bones inward just like a crater. A complicated fracture is one where the bone tears the meninges and leads to bleeding. The fragments can also dislodge and damage the tissues of the brain. If this type of complicated fracture is also an open one, it exposes the meninges and the brain to the environment, increasing the chances of a lethal infection.

Scalp Injuries

Running through the scalp is a large number of arteries and veins which do not retract. This is because of the structure of tissues and damaged blood vessels. This is the reason why cuts to the scalp lead to profuse bleeding. The significant amount of blood lost puts the victim at risk of shock.

Brain Injuries

There are several ways to categorize brain injuries. They can be categorized as acquire or congenital—congenital means existing at or before birth. Congenital brain injuries are injuries that should be handled by some trained medical personnel. Acquired brain injuries are further divided into traumatic and non-traumatic.

Traumatic Brain Injuries

Traumatic brain injuries are often caused by the rapid acceleration of the head like whiplash or a blunt force trauma or hit to the head. This can cause several injuries to the brain and its protective tissue. This can lead to contusions or bruising of the brain tissue, hemorrhage, or hematomas, which is the bleeding in the brain or skull or the stretching and tearing of the brain tissue.

The brain is in a confined and rigid space, so swelling and bleeding will lead to an increase in the intracranial pressure (ICP). The intracranial pressure can lead to a decrease in the perfusion of the brain tissues and herniation of the brain out of the neurocranium. The lack of oxygen and nutrients caused by decreased perfusion can lead to tissue death and permanent brain damage. Short term brain herniation or insufficient perfusion can disturb the normal activities of the brain, causing changes ranging from speech to general cognition. It can also cause damage to the autonomous nervous system, which regulates breathing, blood pressure, and heart rate.

Mild Traumatic Brain Injury

The following symptoms are related to mild traumatic brain injury.

- Altered level of consciousness

- Altered cognition

- Sensory disturbances

- Vomiting and nausea

- General unwellness

Severe Traumatic Brain Injury

The symptoms for a severe traumatic brain injury include those for a mild traumatic brain injury as well as these new symptoms:

- Worsening symptoms of mild traumatic brain injury

- Worsening headaches

- A change in pupil size, even though this is a later developing sign

- Severely altered cognition which includes aphasia, the difficulty in finding and understanding words, slurred speech, paresis, the weakening of one or more limbs, or full-on paralysis.

- Altered vital signs

- Bleeding from the ears

Allergies

An allergy is a response our body gives to foreign substances. These foreign substances are called allergens. These allergens are not typically harmful to our body, but the body recognizes and tags them as invaders and fights to destroy them. These allergens enter the body by various means. They can be swallowed or ingested, inhaled or smelt, injected into the body, or applied on the skin by various means such as medication or insect bite. Allergens include some types of food, pet dander, pollen, molds, dust mites, medication, or animal proteins.

The role of our immune system is to defend the body from harmful substances, and any substance that the body senses as foreign are destroyed. Our immune system reacts when in contact with allergens, although they are not harmful, and may cause inflammation of the skin, airways, sinuses, or digestive system. In severe cases, it can lead to an anaphylactic reaction, which is a life-threatening reaction.

Causes of Allergies

Allergic reactions start when your body mistakes a harmless substance (allergen) for an invader (pathogen) and then produces antibodies to fight them. The antibodies produce a chemical called histamine, which causes allergic symptoms.

- Common allergens include:

- Airborne allergens, such as dust mites, mold spores, animal dander and pollen

- Certain food substances such as peanuts, fish, shellfish, eggs, milk, soy and tree nuts

- Insect stings, such as from a wasp or bee

- Latex

- Nickel and other metals

- Drugs such as penicillin or penicillin-based products.

- Plants such as pollens from grass, weeds, and trees and resins from plants such as poison ivy and poison oak.

- Cosmetics

- Personal care products

Risk Factors for Allergies

Heredity: Children whose parents are allergic to some substances might have the tendency to have those allergies.

- Gender

- Race

- Age

- Exposure to infectious disease during early childhood

- Diet

Symptoms of Allergies

For nasal allergy; such as allergic rhinitis (hay fever), symptoms include runny nose, sneezing, itching of the eyes, nose or roof of the mouth

For allergies of the eyes; such as allergic conjunctivitis, symptoms include redness and itching of the eyes

For allergies of the ears, symptoms include a feeling of fullness, pain and impaired hearing

For allergies in the gastrointestinal tract, symptoms could be vomiting, bloating, abdominal pain, diarrhea

For food allergies; symptoms include tingling in the mouth, swelling of the lips, tongue, face or throat; hives, nausea, fatigue

Symptoms of insect sting allergy include swelling at the site of the sting, itching over the body, cough, wheezing and shortness of breath

Drug allergies cause hives, itchy skin, rash, wheezing

Symptoms of skin allergy include redness and/or peeling of the skin, itchy skin, rashes, eczema, hives

Common Allergic Conditions

Allergic rhinitis (Hay fever): This is one of the most common allergic conditions. It is caused by inhaling allergens such as dust, molds, pollens, or animal dander. It causes irritation of the nose, sneezing, itching, and redness of the eyes. It also leads to inflammation of the cells in the nose, more mucus in the lungs, coughing, wheezing, and shortness of breath.

Asthma: This is a condition where the walls of the airways are inflamed and hypersensitive, which causes the airways to become narrow.

Allergic conjunctivitis: This is the swelling of the tissues that cover the eyeball.

Atopic dermatitis (Eczema): This is a condition where patches of the skin become swollen and itch sometimes.

Hives: This is a skin reaction that causes red, itchy, and raised welts of various sizes and shapes to develop on the skin.

Contact dermatitis: This is the swelling of the skin caused by contact of substances with the skin.

Skin Allergies

Allergies on the skin are common symptoms of allergic reactions. It may be a result of direct contact of the allergens with the skin or triggered by the ingestion of the allergen.

Types of skin allergies:

- Rashes

- Eczema

- Contact dermatitis

- Sore throat

- Hives

- Swollen eyes

- Itching

- Burning

Anaphylaxis

This is a severe, life-threatening allergic reaction. It can affect multiple organs at the same time. Symptoms of anaphylaxis include:

- Loss of consciousness

- Drop-in blood pressure

- Hives and itchy skin

- Shortness of breath

- Nausea

- Vomiting

- Skin rash

- Lightheadedness

- Weak pulse

- Swelling of the tongue or throat

- Nasal congestion, runny nose

- Itchy eyes

- Abdominal discomfort

- Diarrhea

- Coughing and Wheezing

Complications

Anaphylaxis: This occurs as a result of severe allergies. This is mostly triggered by foods, medications, and insect stings.

Asthma: Allergic reactions trigger asthma because these reactions affect the airways and breathing

Sinusitis and infections of the ear and lungs.

Diagnosis

Physical Examination.

Blood test: The manifestation of immunoglobulin E (IgE), an allergy-causing antibody is confirmed for in the blood.

Skin tests: This is usually carried out by an allergist. Different allergens are applied to the skin, and the skin's reaction to these allergens are observed.

Medication

Medications for allergy include:

- Antihistamines

- Corticosteroids

- Decongestants

Another treatment option is immunotherapy. In cases of emergency, an emergency epinephrine shot can be administered.

Prevention

The best prevention of allergies is the avoidance of allergens that lead to reactions.

Asthma

What is Asthma?

Asthma is a condition in which the tube that carries air to your lungs become swollen and narrow. It is a disease that obstructs the flow of air to the lungs. The airways of the lungs are surrounded by smooth muscles and contain mucous glands. The smooth muscles usually contract and relax to control the flow of air into the lungs. The mucous glands defend the airways and trap debris and other cells and take them to the nose to be expelled. In asthma, the muscles of the lungs tighten, swell, and get filled up with mucus because the cells of the airways sense a threat and, in response, produces a lot of mucus. This makes it difficult to breathe. It can also trigger coughing and a whistling sound when breathing.

Asthma is a non-communicable disease. It cannot be transferred by contact from anyone suffering from the disease. Although, it can be transferred from parent to child or caused by environmental factors. Having a parent with asthma is not a guarantee that you would, but there is a tendency that you might develop it.

Asthma cannot be cured, but it can be controlled with treatment. The earlier the treatment, the less its tendency to interrupt your daily activities. With proper management, you can live healthy and active lives.

An asthma attack occurs mostly by the presence of triggers. A trigger is anything that irritates the airways. There are two types of triggers that cause asthma attacks.

Allergic triggers - such as dust mites, pollens, molds, cockroach wastes, pet dander or viral infections

Non-allergic triggers such as smoke, dust, exercise, cold air, air pollutants, or intense emotions.

Symptoms of Asthma

Symptoms of asthma differ in persons. Some exhibit these symptoms only in certain situations such as tedious work, exercise, or presence of triggers, while some exhibit these symptoms all the time.

Signs and symptoms of asthma include:

> **Shortness of breath**: This gives you the feeling that you cannot breathe well and makes it difficult to speak, eat, or sleep.
>
> **Cough**: This often occurs at night or early in the morning. It can also happen at any time of the day. It is common in children.
>
> Increased mucous production: **There is a lot of mucus in the airways because they are swollen**.
>
> **Chest pain or tightness**: This is an unpleasant feeling caused by the pressure of the extra fluid in the lungs

Wheezing: This is the whistling sound produced when breathing out. This is common in children.

Trouble sleeping as a result of shortness of breath or coughing.

Associated symptoms include lightheadedness, palpitations, and fatigue. The onset of new symptoms includes aging or lack of response to appropriate medications.

Causes of Asthma

Researchers have been unable to determine the cause of asthma, but certain risk factors have been associated with asthma.

Asthma could result from interactions between a person's genetics and interactions with the environment.

Risk factors for asthma include:

Family history: Children with parents that have asthma are more likely to develop asthma.

Gender: Asthma is said to occur more frequently in boys than in girls. Experts have said that the size of a young male's airways is smaller in comparison to a young female's.

Allergies: These are immune reactions triggered by allergens. People with allergies are more likely to develop asthma. This is not to say that everyone who has an allergy will develop asthma or that everyone who has asthma is affected by allergens.

Atopy: This is a genetic condition where one tends to develop eczema, hay fever (allergic rhinitis), or allergic conjunctivitis. It causes increased sensitivity to common allergens that should not affect the body.

Obesity: Accumulation of fat around the chest might squeeze the lungs and make it more difficult to breathe. The fat tissues also produce inflammatory substances that might influence the lungs and trigger asthma.

Environment: Air pollution, toxic gases, fumes from exhaust pipes of generators, engines and vehicles, cold temperature, high humidity, and other indoor sources of air pollutants can trigger asthma.

Smoking: Smoking appears to lower lung functions, and this makes one more susceptible to asthma

Premature birth: Children born before 37 weeks might be at greater risk of developing asthma.

Lung infections: Infants and children who develop lung infections at an early age might be at the risk of developing asthma. Viral respiratory illness, such as a respiratory syncytial virus (RSV), might cause asthma.

Hormones: Hormonal imbalances during or after menopause might lead to the development of asthma.

Occupational exposures: Exposure to dust particles, gases, chemical fumes, and vapor at the workplace can cause asthma.

Types of Asthma

Allergic asthma: This occurs as a result of allergies or existing allergic conditions such as hay fever (allergic rhinitis) in the individual. This causes hypersensitivity and inflammation of the cells in the airways of the individual and other symptoms of asthma.

Exercise-induced asthma: This type of asthma is triggered by exercise or physical exertion. This makes it difficult to breathe, and other symptoms of asthma, such as coughing and wheezing, might occur.

Cough-variant asthma: The major symptom of this type of asthma is severe coughing. Triggers are usually respiratory infections and exercise.

Occupational asthma: This is asthma that results from workplace triggers.

Nocturnal (nighttime) asthma: In this type of asthma, chances of having symptoms are increased at night time. Asthma is influenced by sleep-wake cycles. This may be triggered by increased exposure to allergens, cooling of the airways, reclining position, or hormone secretions.

Classification of Asthma

Asthma can vary from very mild symptoms to severe and life-treating cases. Classification of asthma include:

Mild intermittent asthma: Symptoms of this kind are usually mild and do not often occur, mostly exercise-induced asthma. These symptoms include coughing, swollen airways, mucus in the airways, and wheezing. One would usually only need a rescue inhaler to manage this kind of asthma. Medications will be determined by how severe attacks are when they occur. People at risk of this kind of asthma include those with a family history, smokers, those with obesity or allergies, and those exposed to pollution.

Mild persistent asthma: Symptoms of mild persistent asthma are mild but occur more often. Individuals are advised to avoid substances that trigger attacks and might be placed on low-dose inhaled corticosteroid medication.

Moderate persistent asthma: Symptoms of asthma occur more frequently, probably once each day. A higher dose of inhaled corticosteroids may be prescribed.

Severe persistent asthma: Symptoms of asthma repeatedly occur within a day. There is a lesser response to treatment in these cases. Such individuals would be prescribed more aggressive treatment and medication combinations.

Diagnosis of Asthma

Several tests may be conducted to diagnose asthma.

Physical examination: This includes an examination of the nose, throat, and upper airways, breathing sounds, and signs of allergic conditions on the skin.

Spirometry: This is a test used to check lung function and used to diagnose lung conditions such as asthma and Chronic Obstructive Lung Disease (COPD). The spirometer is used to measure the amount of air a person can breathe in a second, and the total volume of air that can be exhaled in one forced breath.

Exhaled nitric oxide test: High levels of nitric oxide in breath indicate the airways are inflamed.

Peak Flow Meter test: This measures the fastest speed at which you can exhale air from your lungs after taking a deep breath. If the airways are inflamed, the peak flow levels will be lower.

TREATMENT OF ASTHMA

Medications for asthma include rescue inhalers, inhaled corticosteroids, and long-acting bronchodilators. Combination of long-acting bronchodilators and inhaled corticosteroids are very effective and used in severe cases.

Burns

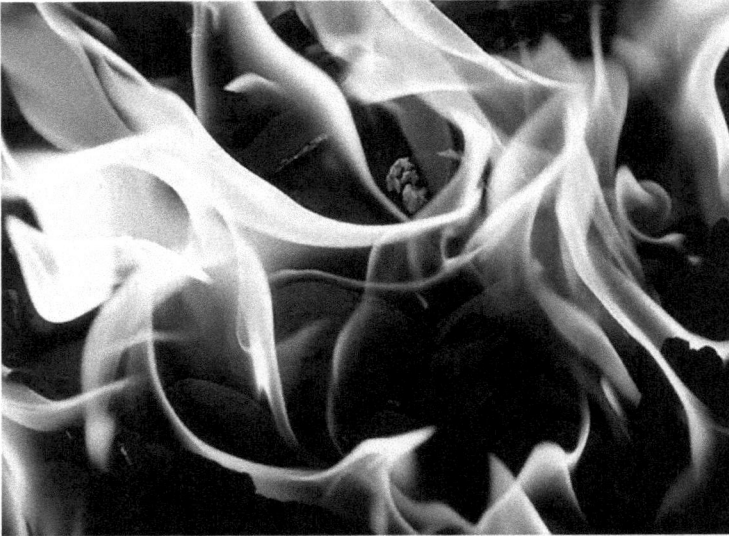

A burn is damage to the tissues of the skin caused by heat, overexposure to the sun, cold, chemicals, electricity, friction, or radiation. Burns vary from minor injuries to life-threatening emergency situations. Burns cause the affected skin cells to die. The cause and degree of injury determine the kind of treatment to be given.

Causes of Burns

Cause of burn include:

- Hot liquid or steam

- Fire

- Hot metal, glass or other objects

- Radiation

- Sunlight or ultraviolet rays

- Electrical currents

- Chemicals

- Abuse

Types of Burns

Friction burns: These are caused by the movement of hard objects on the surface of the skin.

Cold burns: These are also called frostbites. It occurs when the skin is in contact with cold objects for a prolonged time or in freezing temperatures,

Thermal burns: These are caused by contact of the skin with very hot objects. Hot fluids, flames, and steam can cause thermal burns.

Radiation burns: Exposure to the sun and other sources of radiation such as x-rays or radiation therapy may cause radiation burns. Sunburn is an example of radiation burn.

Chemical burns: These occur when strong acids, detergents, or solvents touch the skin.

Electrical burns: Contact of the skin with electrical current causes electrical burns.

Degree of Burns

First degree burns: These are also called superficial burns. They affect the outer layer of the skin. They appear red without blisters. The pain usually doesn't last more than three days. There could be minor swelling and peeling of the skin as the burn heals. Treatment for first-degree burns such as using an antibiotic ointment, taking pain relief drugs, or applying the cream to soothe the pain can be done at home.

Second degree burns: These burns affect the outer layer of the skin and the layer beneath it. It can cause swelling and redness of the skin, severe pain, and blisters when healing begins. Deep second degree burns may cause scarring. Healing usually takes longer.

Third-degree burns: These burns affect the layers of the skin and the fat layer beneath the skin. The burned areas may appear black, brown, or white. The skin texture becomes leathery. In third-degree burns, pain is often not felt because of nerve damage. Treatments of such burns might require surgery.

Fourth-degree burns: These injuries usually destroy all layers of the skin and affect deeper tissues such as muscle, tendons, or bone.

Complications

All burns have the risk of infections. Severe complications are usually associated with third-degree burns. These complications include:

- A bacterial infection which may lead to sepsis; an infection of the blood.

- Tetanus: This is a bacterial infection that affects the nervous system, leading to problems with contractions.

- Hypovolemia: This is low blood volume as a result of fluid loss

- Hypothermia: Low body temperature

- Keloids: Overgrowth of scar tissue leads to scars

- Contractures: These include bone and joint problems caused by the shortening and tightening of the skins, muscles, and tendons.

Treatment

Treatment to be administered on burns depend on the intensity of the injury. Medications that can help healing include:

- Pain and anxiety medications

- Burn creams and ointments

- Intravenous fluid to prevent dehydration and organ failure

- Antibiotics

- Tetanus toxoids

- Dressing

Other treatment options include physical therapy, skin grafts, and plastic surgery. These are usually required in severe cases.

Prevention

In order to reduce cases of household burns:

- Put hot fluids away from the reach of children and pets

- Keep all electrical appliances away from water and other liquids

- Unplug electrical appliances when not in use

- Cover unused electrical outlets

- Wear protective clothing when handling chemicals

- Keep a fire extinguisher handy

- Use protective wears when handling hot objects

- Avoid peak sunlight

Concussion

What is Concussion?

A concussion is a mild injury to the brain caused by a blow to the head or violent shaking of the head and body. Effects of concussion include headache, problems with concentration, memory, balance, and coordination. These effects are usually temporary but might sometimes lead to unconsciousness.

Concussions can be caused mostly by fall and collision during sporting activities.

Causes of Concussion

A concussion is caused by a violent blow to the head, neck, or upper body. The brain is usually cushioned by cerebrospinal fluid, but a sudden jolt can cause your brain to move back and forth in your skull. This affects brain function, mostly for just a short period of time. Sometimes, these injuries can lead to bleeding in the brain, which could be fatal.

Risk Factors for Concussion

Factors that increase the chances of concussion include:

- A fall

- Sports activities such as football, hockey, rugby, boxing, and other contact sport

- Accidents

- Physical abuse

- Combat

- Previous concussions

Symptoms of Concussion

A concussion may present itself immediately after an injury or may not form for several hours, days, weeks, or months even after the said injury.

The common signs of a concussion, especially after an injury, are memory loss, chronic headaches, and confusion. The victim may have no recollection of the events leading to the concussion.

Symptoms of a concussion are

- Headaches

- Ringing ears

- Queasiness

- Unsettled stomach

- Weariness

- Blurry vision

- Dizziness

- Slurred speech

- Amnesia

- Temporary loss of consciousness

- Sleep disturbances

- Irritability

- Sensitivity to light and noise

- Disorders of taste and smell

- Confusion

- Concussions may be accompanied by injuries to the spine, especially during accidents.

Concussion in Babies

Some common signs of concussion in babies include:

- Vomiting

- Drainage from the mouth, ears, and nose

- Irritability

- Drowsiness

- Loss of balance and unsteady walking

- Seizures

- Excessive crying

Types of Concussions

A concussion can vary from mild to severe, depending on how long the symptoms get resolved.

Mild concussion: This is also called Grade 1 concussion. Symptoms usually last for less than 15 minutes. There is no loss of consciousness.

Moderate concussion: Grade 2 concussion does not cause loss of consciousness, but symptoms do last longer than 15 minutes.

Severe concussion: In severe (Grade 3) concussion, there is the loss of consciousness, sometimes just for a few seconds.

Complications

Complications of concussion include:

- **Post-traumatic headaches**: Persistence of headaches for days after injury

- **Post-traumatic vertigo**: A sense of dizziness for days, weeks or even months after injury

- **Post-concussion syndrome**: Persistence of concussion symptoms beyond three weeks after the injury

- **Cumulative effects of multiple brain injuries**: Effects of repeated head injuries

- **Second impact syndrome**: An experience of a second concussion before symptoms of a first injury have resolved may lead to brain swelling. This can be fatal to the brain.

Diagnosis

- **Physical Examination**: This involves the examination of the head and parts of the body that the injury occurred.

- **MRI scan**: This is done to check for injuries in the brain

- **Electroencephalogram**: This monitors brain waves. This is done mostly in cases of seizures.

- **Special eye test**: This involves the assessment of visual changes such as changes in pupil size, eye movements, and light sensitivity.

Treatment

The treatment of concussion depends on how severe the symptoms are. Most times, no major medication is administered, except for headaches where pain relievers are prescribed. Victims are advised to get enough rest, avoid sports and other strenuous activities and alcohol.

In severe cases such as bleeding in the brain, swelling of the brain, or a serious injury to the brain, surgery might be required.

Prevention

To prevent or minimize head injuries, the following should be practiced.

- Wear protective gears during sports and other recreational activities

- Use a seat belt while driving

- Avoid wet or slippery floors

- Exercise regularly. This helps improve balance

- Avoid dark places. Keep the house well lit to help prevent falls.

Tendons and Fractures

Tendons

Tendons, which are sinew in a tough tissue, connect muscles to bones. They are very strong and can withstand a great deal of tension. They are mostly made up of specialized fiber cells known as tenocytes. These tenocytes produce collagen molecules that gather to form the collagen fibrils. Those collagen fibrils then gather to form what is known as the extracellular matrix of the tendons.

These extracellular matrixes then lie parallel to each other and organize into bundles. The endotendineum binds the bundles. The endotendineum, which is a loose connective tissue, is also made up of collagen fibrils and elastic fibers. The bundles of extracellular matrixes are then bound by the epitenon, which is a sheath of dense irregular connective tissue. The fascia then covers the whole tendon. The space between the fascia and the tendon is filled with a fatty areolar tissue called the paratenon. The Sharpey's fibers are what hold the tendons and bones together.

The cells of the tendon communicate to each other by gap junctions. This enables them to detect and respond to mechanical loading. The blood vessels of the tendon lie parallel to the collagen fibers in the endotenon. Nerve endings are absented in the endotenon but present in the paratenon and epitenon.

The length of tendon varies from person to person. Tendon length decides the actual and potential size of the muscles. It is determined by genetics, and there has been no proven effect of the environment on the tendon length.

Functions

The tendons are mechanisms by which the muscles connect to bones. They transmit the force produced by the muscles, controlling locomotion, and providing stability for the skeletal structure.

Some tendons possess elastic properties and function as springs. These tendons are called energy-storing tendons. They store elastic energy to be released later in the movement of the muscles. Also, the ability of the tendon to stretch allows the muscles to function with less or no change in length, generating greater force.

Injuries of the Tendon

Strain: This is an overstretch or tearing of the tendon. Common parts of the body where strain occurs are the leg, foot, and back. Strains usually occur as a result of habitual movements and athletics. Symptoms of a strain include pain and swelling in the affected area. The affected area may feel warm to touch.

Tendonitis: This also occurs as a result of the overuse of the tendon. Symptoms of tendonitis include pain when the muscle is moved and swelling of the area. Deep

Treatment

Treatment for strain include:

- **Rest**: Immobilization of the injured part aids healing. Immobilization braces and clutches may be used, if necessary.

- **Ice**: A wrap of ice in a towel helps to soothe the pain and allows the tendon to relax

- **Compression**: The use of a compression bandage helps to reduce swelling

- **Elevation**: The injured part should be placed above the heart to reduce swelling and aid healing

- **Medication**: Anti-inflammatory and pain relief drugs could be administered to help reduce pain and swelling.

Prevention

- Warm-up before exercising

- Start slowly and build gradually

- Maintain a healthy weight

- Rest. Take a day off after an intense exercise or strenuous activity

- Wear shoes that fit well

- Observe and listen to your body

- Stretch your body

Fractures

The skeletal framework of the body is made up of bones. The bones are sites for attachment of muscles, which allows them to move and perform activities. The bones also serve as a shield for the organs and partake in the production of blood cells.

A complete or partial break in the bone is known as a fracture. The fracture of bones varies from mild to severe. It may be a result of a strong impact, stress, or mild traumatic injury. It can also occur due to medical conditions that weaken the bones such as osteoporosis, osteopenia, or bone cancer. Fractures are commonly caused by car accidents, falls, sports activities.

Symptoms

- Swelling, bruising and tenderness around the injury

- Intense pain

- Numbness and tingling feeling at the affected area

- Discolored skin around the affected area

- Deformity - the bone shifts out of its place

- Problem moving the injured part

- Bleeding

Types of Fractures

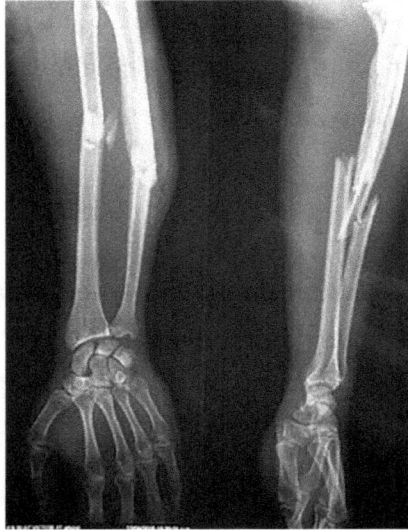

Closed fracture: This type of fracture does not break through the skin or damage surrounding tissues.

Open fracture: This is also known as a compound fracture. The fracture damages the surrounding tissues and breaks through the skin. There is a tendency to develop a deep bone infection.

Avulsion fracture: This occurs as a result of a muscle or ligament pulling on a bone, thereby causing it to fracture.

Comminuted fracture: In this type of fracture, the bone is broken into many pieces

Compression fracture: This occurs in the spongy bone in the spine, where a part of the vertebra collapses

Fracture dislocation: In fracture-dislocation, a joint in the body becomes dislocated and one of the bones of the joint breaks.

Greenstick fracture: This is an incomplete break in the bone because the other part of the bone can bend. This is common in children with softer and more elastic bones.

Torus fracture: This is the deformation of the bones without cracking. It is common in children and usually painful.

Impacted fracture: In this type of fracture, a fragment of the broken bone goes into another bone

Intraarticular fracture: In fractures like this, there is an extension of the break into the surface of the joint.

Longitudinal fracture: The fracture occurs along the length of the bone.

Oblique fracture: The fracture occurs diagonally to the axis of the bone

Spiral fracture: This is a fracture where one part of the bone has been twisted.

Transverse fracture: This is a straight break across the bone.

Pathological fracture: This is as a result of an underlying disease or condition that weakened the bone.

Hairline fracture: This is a partial break of the bone, and it is usually difficult to detect initially.

Complications

The severity of a fracture depends on the type of fracture and its location in the body. Complications of fractures can be divided into three

Immediate complications: This occurs at the time of the fracture. Symptoms include hypovolemic shock; injury at major blood vessels, muscles and tendons, joints and viscera

Early complications: This occurs in the first few days after the fracture. Symptoms include pulmonary syndrome, fat embolism syndrome, sepsis, deep vein thrombosis, infection.

Late complications: This occurs a long while after the fracture. Symptoms include shortening, joint stiffness, osteoarthritis.

Diagnosis

- Physical examination

- X-ray tests

- MRI scans

Treatment

Bone healing is a process that occurs naturally. Treatment is given to ensure the maximal function of the affected area after healing. The ends of the broken bones require to be aligned for the healing process to begin.

Treatment includes:

- Immobilization: The bones need to stay aligned for it to heal. Objects such as plaster casts, metal plates and screws, intramedullary nails, and external fixators can be used to hold the bones in place.

- Physical therapy

- Surgery

Prevention

Nutrition: The body requires calcium to keep the bones healthy and strong. Sources of calcium include milk, yogurt, cheese, and dark leafy vegetables.

Sunlight: The sunlight is a source of vitamin D, which helps our body to absorb calcium. Other sources of vitamin D are eggs and fish oil.

Physical activity: The bones get stronger from performing weight-bearing exercises. These exercises include skipping, walking, jumping, running, and dancing.

Chapter 3

The First Aid Kit

First aid kits are essential that should be in every home and workplace because they are always used at one point or the other. There are also first aid kits that have been made commercially available for sale at several retail shops or chain stores. What you need out of the first aid box depends on your level of medical training and how far away help is.

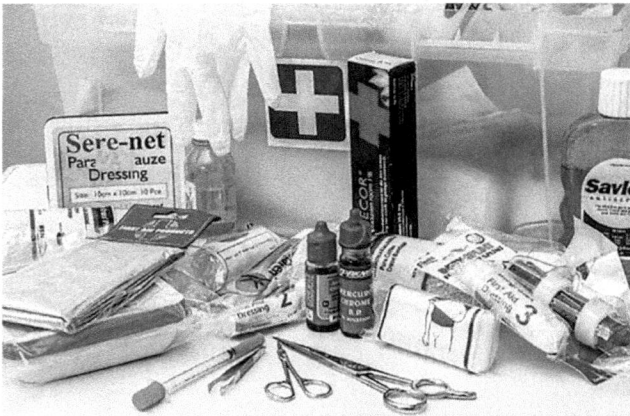

The basics which must be included in a home and travel first aid kit include the supplies that are often used to treat minor traumatic injuries such as:

- Burns

- Abrasions and scrapes

- Cuts

- Splinters

- Stings

- Strains

- Sprains

A comprehensive first aid kit is important for travel, especially when going to areas that are far from medical centers. Within the kit should be personal medical items like allergy drugs and other common items that can be used to less common symptoms of viral respiratory illnesses like fever, cough, nasal congestion, or sore throat. Within the first aid kit should also be supplied that can take care of ailments like cuts, mild pain, skin problems, allergies, gastrointestinal problems, and so on.

A first aid kit does not have to be bulky. It can be a simple kit by filling it with items that have several uses. Any bag-like item that offers a good view of the interior can serve as a household first aid kit.

Kits that are packed for travel or those stored in the car should be drop-proof and water-resistant. Several items can serve this purpose, like a personal kit, a fanny pack, or a makeup bag. Household items like oven bags or resealable sandwich bags can also serve as a first aid kit.

The first aid kit should be inspected twice a year or more, and all expired drugs replaced immediately. The kitchen is the smartest place to put a home kit, not just because it is the hub of every home where most family activities take place but also because the kitchen is an airy place. The humidity of the bathroom will quickly reduce the shelf life of the items in the first aid kit.

The travel first aid kit should be within reach, depending on the activities planned for the trip, either in the luggage or the bag. First aid kits designed for everyday use should remain in the car. Places, where long periods of time are spent like the travel trailer, the vacation homes, the boats, the cabins, and so on, should all have their individual first aid kits.

First Aid Kit Essentials

The following items should be included in your first aid kit. They can all be bought at the local, well-packed drug store and you can also inquire from the pharmacist the best items to stock.

Included in the home kit should be:

- Adhesive tape

- Anesthetic spray or lotion

- Sterile gauze pads

- Ace bandages

- Adhesive bandages

- Oral antihistamines

- Topical corticosteroids

- Aloe vera topical gel or cream

- Exam gloves

- Polysporin antibiotic cream

- Non-adhesive pads

- Pocket masks for CPR

- Resealable oven bags. Can be used to hold contaminated articles or as an ice pack

- Safety pins - used to remove splinters and hold triangular bandage slings in place.

- Scissors

- Triangular bandages which can be used as a tourniquet, a sling, or a towel.

- Tweezers which is used for splinters, stingers, or tick removal.

Travel Kits

The following items should be included in a travel kit.

- Adhesive tape

- Sterile gauze pads

- Antacids for indigestion

- Antidiarrheal

- Antihistamine cream

- Antiseptic agents for cleaning wounds and hands

- Aspirin for mild pain and heart attacks

- Adhesive bandages of all sizes

- Diphenhydramine or loratadine

- Topical corticosteroids

- Aloe vera topical cream or gel for burn relief

- A book on first aid

- A cigarette lighter can be used to sterilize instruments and start a fire to keep warm or create a signal for help

- Cough medications

- Dental kits

- Exam gloves

- A flashlight

- Ibuprofen

- Insect repellant

- A knife, preferably a small Swiss Army type

- Moleskin which is often applied to blisters or hot spots

- Nasal spray decongestants for nasal congestion from allergies or cold

- Non-adhesive wound pads

- Polysporin antibiotic ointment

- Plastic resealable bags

- Pocket masks for CPR

- Safety pins

- Scissors

- Sunscreen

- Tweezers

Chapter 4

First Aid Treatment for
Health Emergencies and Conditions.

In this chapter, we will finally describe how to apply first aid treatment and practices for emergency health situations. One major thing to keep in mind when applying these procedures is ALWAYS to remain calm and ask for CONSENT. This book covers a wide variety of situations you might find yourself or a loved one in. Here goes.

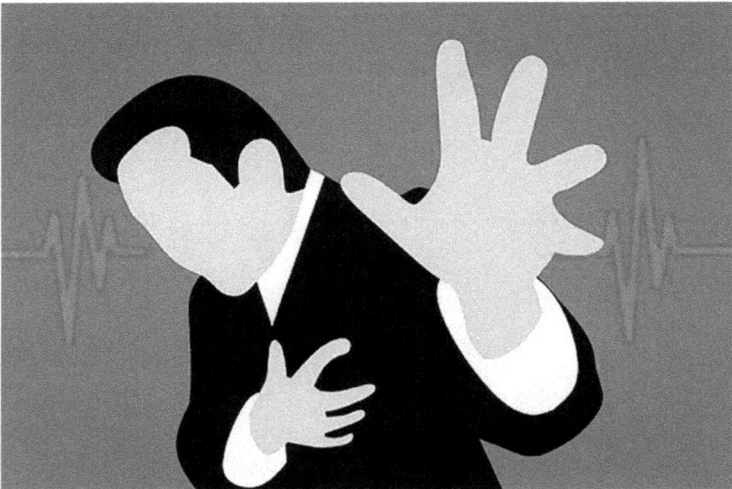

First Aid Treatment during a Heart Attack

The main sign of a heart attack is insistent chest discomfort that goes away and then comes back or lasts for more than 3 to 5 minutes. If you see that a person is experiencing the symptoms of a heart attack, then it is best to call the local emergency services immediately. A person can be experiencing a heart attack and still categorically deny the symptoms are that serious. Do not let this deter you, especially if you are sure. Once you believe a person is experiencing a heart attack, it is smart you act immediately.

Heart attacks can easily lead to cardiac arrests, and cardiac arrests can easily lead to death, but this added damage to the heart can be prevented by immediate action. This makes it important to act immediately; you notice the signs of a heart attack in anyone. Most of the deaths that happen due to heart attacks occur within 2 hours of the first signal. A whole lot of them could have been saved if the victims recognized their symptoms for what it was and acted accordingly, or those who were present when it happens had acted quickly.

Several people who experience attack attacks dilly-dally in getting medical care, waiting for the symptoms to dissipate. When it refuses to go away, then they find their way to get care. The average person waits 2 hours before going to the hospital. The damage caused to the heart can be reduced even in the aftermath of a heart attack by early treatment with the proper medications. These medications are usually most effective when given within the first hour of the heart attack signals.

If you observe or suspect that someone is experiencing a heart attack, then you should do the following:

- Call the local emergency number immediately.

- Stop whatever the person is doing and have the victim rest comfortably. By resting, the need of the heart for oxygen will reduce greatly. Those who are experiencing a heart attack can breathe easier when in a sitting position.

- Loosen any uncomfortable or tight clothing that they may have on.

- Observe the victim closely for any changes in appearance or behavior until the trained medical personnel take over.

- If the victim loses consciousness or stops breathing, then you need to perform CPR and or use an AED if one is available.

- Be sure to ask the victim if he or she has a history of any heart disease. Some of those who have heart disease have prescribed medication for their chest pain. You can get the medication and help the victim take the needed medication.

- Remember to be calm and comforting. This will go a long way in reducing the anxiety and discomfort of the victim.

- Talk to the victim, if possible, and the onlookers to derive as much information as you can about the victim.

- You can also offer aspirin as medical protocols, and local protocols allow. Be sure that the victim can swallow. Make sure the victim has not been instructed to avoid aspirin by his or her health care provider. Also, make sure that the victim does not have any known contraindications to aspirin.

- Do not try to take the victim to the hospital yourself. Wait instead for the medical personnel because the victim's condition might rapidly deteriorate on the way.

Aspirin to Reduce Heart Attack Damage

Whenever the victim is showing early signs of a heart attack, you can help a said victim while he or she is still conscious. You can offer him or her the right doses of aspirin when the symptoms begin. That does not mean you should dally in reaching out to the local emergency services, as that is the most important way to help a person who is suffering from a heart attack. You should help the victim into a comfortable position before offering the aspirin. As the victim is still conscious and can take the aspirin orally, you should inquire about the following things from the victim.

- Do you have any stomach diseases or a stomach ulcer?

- Do you take any blood thinners like warfarin?

- Are you allergic to aspirin?

- Have you been instructed by your doctors to avoid aspirin?

If the answer to all those questions is no, then, and only then can you offer the victim two chewable baby aspirins of 81 mg each or one adult, 325 mg of an adult aspirin tablet, and some water. Ensure not to offer aspirin coated products or aspirin products that are meant for other or multiple uses like fever, headaches, or cold.

You must be offering only aspirin and not acetaminophen, Tylenol, or nonsteroidal anti-inflammatory drugs (NSAIDs) like Aleve, Advil, ibuprofen, Motrin, or naproxen.

First Aid Treatment for Cardiac Arrest

Cardiac arrests are sudden, occurring without prior warning and manifesting as a heart attack. The suddenness of cardiac arrest accounts for over 300,000 deaths annually in the United States alone. The irregular and disorderly electrical activity of the heart leads to sudden cardiac arrests. Medically, it is termed arrhythmias. The most common form of arrhythmias is ventricular fibrillation, also known as V-fib.

The Cardiac Chain of Survival

To save someone who is suffering from a cardiac arrest, CPR alone might not do the trick. That is why it is important to get advanced medical personnel on the ground as soon as possible. The chain of survival is what presents the best chance of survival for a victim who is suffering from a sudden cardiac arrest.

- Immediate recognition and early access to emergency medical services. The sooner someone figures out what is wrong and alerts the proper authorities, the sooner the EMS personnel arrive and take over.

- Immediate CPR is the next step. It is not enough to recognize and call the emergency services; someone must perform CPR on the victim. CPR helps in supplying blood to the brain and vital organs. Without the supply of blood to those organs, they begin to die, and this can cause lasting damage should the victim survive. The immediate application of CPR would help keep the victim alive until the medical personnel arrives or an AED is made available.

- Immediate defibrillation, which is an electric shock to the heart, can help to restore the heart's rhythm.

- Immediate advanced medical care is the last on the chain of survival. The EMS personnel will give the much-needed advanced medical care and move the victim to the hospital.

Any and every delay of CPR and defibrillation reduces the chances of survival of the victim by 10 percent. The chain of survival is interdependent, relying on its other links to function efficiently. Taking quick action and following the survival chain helps the odds of the patient to survive a cardiac arrest. As the first link on the chain of survival, it is important you call the police immediately you observe that the victim, whoever he or she may be, young or old, is not breathing and is unconscious. While waiting for help to arrive, you need to perform CPR to increase the victim's chances of survival.

Cpr and Defibrillation

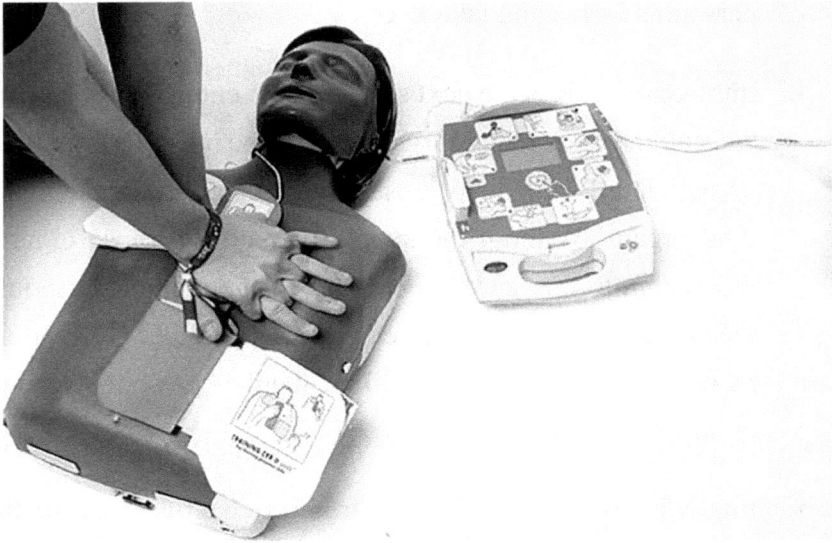

While waiting for help to arrive, the best course of action is to perform immediate CPR as well as defibrillation. That allows the cells of the brain and other organs to continue to have the oxygen they need to continue living for a short time before all the oxygen in the blood is used up. CPR involves a sequence of chest compressions and rescue breaths. As the heart is not beating, the chest compressions would help in circulating the blood having oxygen. The chest compressions, given together with rescue breaths, do the work of the heart and the lungs and increase the chances of survival for the victim.

That does not mean that the CPR alone is enough to get the job done. There are instances when performing CPR is not enough to correct the underlying problems of the heart. In cases like that, an AED delivers defibrillation. The electric shock given by defibrillation is enough to interfere with the heart's electric activates just long enough for the heart to spontaneously develop the right and effective rhythm, all on its own. Early CPR and early defibrillation greatly increase the chances of survival for a cardiac arrest patient.

How to Perform CPR for Adults

Not everyone needs CPR. To decide if an unconscious adult requires CPR, there are emergency procedures that need to be followed.

- Check the victim as well as the scene

- Call for help or the local emergency services.

- Check for the victim's breathing for no more than 10 seconds

- Check quickly for severe bleeding

- If the victim is not breathing, begin CPR immediately.

To ensure effective chest compressions, the victim's back must be on a firm and flat surface. If the victim is on a soft surface like a bed or a sofa, quickly transfer the victim to a firm and flat surface like the floor before you begin compressions.

In order to begin compressions on an adult, you need to position your body correctly, and you do that by kneeling directly beside the victim's upper chest. The correct hand placement ensures that your arms and elbows are as straight as possible to ensure your shoulders are directly over your hands. The position of your body as a first aider is very important to give effective chest compressions. Because you need the necessary depth in order to compress the victim's chest straight down, making use of the correct body position will make it less tiresome for you. This is very helpful, especially when you are the only one available to help the victim.

The correct hand position is to place the heel of one hand on the victim's sternum or breast bone. That is at the center of his or her chest. You then place your other hand directly on top of the first hand. Try to keep your fingers away from the chest. You can do this by either holding the fingers upward or interlacing them. If you feel the notch that is at the end of the sternum, then move your hands slightly upwards.

Individuals with arthritis in hand can still perform CPR on an unconscious victim by clasping the wrist of the hand, which is positioned on the chest with the freehand. Ensure that the person's clothing does not interfere with you finding the right-hand position or disturb, in any way, your ability to give efficient compressions. If in any way, it does, the clothes need to be removed or loosened so as to allow for deep compressions in the center of the victim's chest.

Make sure you push hard and fast to give a rate of at least 100 chest compressions per minute. 100 chest compressions per minute refer to the speed of the compressions and not the number of the compressions that are given per minute. While compressing the chest, it would help if you counted out loud until you have reached 30 chest compressions. Pushing down while saying the number and releasing at the word 'and' will help you keep a nice and steady rhythm while compressing.

Compressions should be given by pushing the sternum downward by at least 2 inches. The upward and downward movement of the sternum should be a smooth one and not a jerky one. Be sure to push straight down the sternum with all the weight of your upper body and not just with your arm muscles. The weight of your upper body will provide the force you need to compress the chest. Do not compress the chest in a rocking motion. Rocking back and forth is a less efficient compression that only wastes the effort of the first aider. Easily tiring arms and shoulders is indications of poor and incorrect body position.

With each compression, release the pressure without changing hand positions or removing your hands. Only when the chest returns to its normal position can you compress the chest again. Do not stop the compressions and maintain a steady down and up motion. Half of the time should be spent pushing down while the other half is spent coming up. Pressing down means squeezing the walls of the heart together and forcing blood to go out of the heart. By coming up and relieving the pressure, the chambers of the heart fills up with blood.

Once 30 chest compressions have been given, the airway should be opened using a head-tilt/chin-lift technique to give 2 rescue breaths. The rescue breaths must clearly make the chest rise and should only last for about one second. The rescue breath technique is:

- Open up the airway and give rescue breaths, one after the other.

- Make sure the head is tilted back, and the chin is lifted.

- The nose should be pinched shut to make a complete seal over the victim's mouth.

- Blow into the victim's mouth for only a second and ensure that the chest clearly rises.

The cycle of chest compressions and rescue breaths should then continue until help arrives. Try to avoid any interruptions to the chest compressions. Every cycle of chest compressions and rescue breaths should only take about 24 seconds.

Should responders trained at CPR are available at the scene with the victim, they should identify themselves as trained people. While one of them begins chest compressions, the other one should reach out to the local emergency services for help. Should the responder performing chest compressions be tired, the other one can take over.

There are only a handful of situations when CPR can be stopped. Those situations include:

- When there is an obvious sign of life like breathing.

- When an AED is available and ready for use.

- When there is trained personnel or EMS responder who is ready to take over.

- When the scene becomes unsafe.

- When you are too exhausted to take over.

Should you notice at any time that the victim is breathing, you can stop the CPR. Ensure to keep the airway open and continue to monitor the victim's breathing for any changes in condition until the trained EMS personnel can take over.

Cardiac Emergencies in Infants and Children

While children and infants hardly suffer from a cardiac emergency, it does happen, often on the heels of a respiratory emergency. The causes of cardiac arrest in children and infants are often due to:

- Breathing or airway problems.

- An accident or a traumatic injury.

- Congenital heart disease.

- A hard blow to the chest

- Sudden infant death syndrome (SIDS)

Just like any adult, should you notice a child or an infant is not breathing, then perform CPR immediately. The principles of CPR for an adult, chest compressions, and rescue breaths, are also the same for a child or an infant. The only difference, though, is that the techniques for CPR are different in infants and children as a result of their smaller bodies.

CPR for a Child

For an unconscious child who is not breathing, place the child on a flat and firm surface face-up. Just like an adult, you locate the proper hand position by placing the heel of your hand on the breastbone. Move your hand slightly upwards if you feel the notch of the sternum. The position is also the same, kneeling right next to the upper chest of the child and positioning your shoulders over your hands while keeping your arms and elbows as straight as possible.

30 chest compressions are given, hard, and fast to a 2-inch depth and at a rate of 100 compressions per minute. Remember to lift up and allow the chest to expand to its normal position before compressing, but remember not to change hand positions. The airway should be opened after the 30 compressions to give 2 rescue breaths. Each rescue breath ought to last a second but should be enough to make the chest rise clearly. The head-tilt/chin-lift technique should also be used to open the airway of the child victim.

Just as an adult, CPR does not stop unless one of the following happens:

- There are obvious signs of life like breathing.

- An AED is available and ready to use

- There is another trained responder or EMS personnel who can take over

- You are too tired to continue.

- The area becomes unsafe.

Should you see a change in the breathing pattern of the child, hold CPR, keep the airway open, and watch out for any changes in the child's condition until the EMS personnel take over.

CPR for Infants

To begin CPR for an infant, you must first find the right position for compressions. One hand must be kept on the infant's forehead in order to maintain an open airway. The pads of two or three fingers of the available hand are then used to compress the center of the chest just below the nipple line towards the feet. Again, if the notch at the end of the infant's sternum is felt, move the fingers slightly up towards the head.

30 chest compressions should be given with the pads of the fingers, compressing the chest about 1 and a half inches. The compressions, while hard and fast, must not be jerky but smooth. Make sure you keep a steady rhythm, and there are no pauses during each compression. Do not release your fingers from its position on the infant victim's chest when the fingers are coming up. The compressions should take place at the rate of 100 compressions per minute. 2 rescue breaths should be given after 30 compressions. Each rescue breath should cover the infant victim's nose and mouth, last for only a second, and should clearly make the chest rise.

The cycle of 40 chest compressions and 2 rescue breaths continues except in any of these situations:

- There are obvious signs of life like breathing.

- An AED is available for use

- You can no longer continue due to fatigue

- There is another responder able and ready to take over

- The scene is not safe.

Should you observe that the infant is breathing on his or her own, stop the CPR immediately, ensure to keep the airway open, and continue monitoring the breathing. Watch out for any changes in the infant's condition until the EMS personnel are available and ready to take over.

In times when the chest does not rise with the initial rescue breath, tilt the head back again before giving the second breath. If the second breath does not do the trick, then the victim might be choking. If, after successive compressions and rescue breaths, there is no change in the chest movement, look around for any object that might be obstructing the airway. If you see any, remove it.

If there are reasons you are unwilling or unable to perform a full CPR with rescue breaths, then give continuous chest compressions. Only do so once you have checked the scene for any immediate danger, checked out the victim to rule out any other underlying injuries, and reached out to the local emergency services. The chest compressions should continue until the EMS personnel arrive on the scene, or the victim shows signs of life like breathing.

Automated External Defibrillator

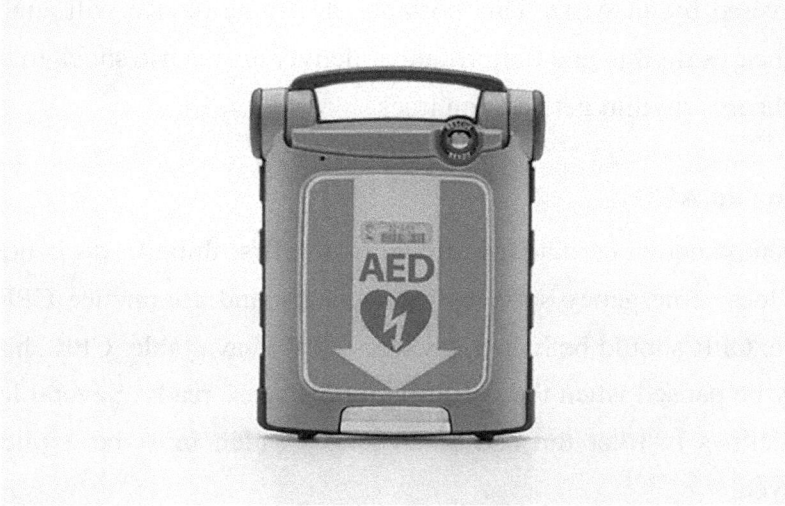

When there is a problem in the heart due to injury or disease, the signals that tell the heart to pump blood are disrupted, leading to abnormal heart rhythm that can interrupt the heart's ability to pump blood. The most common type of these interruptions which cause a cardiac arrest is called ventricular fibrillation. It happens when the ventricles of the heart fibrillate or quiver without an organized rhythm, and the electrical impulses all fire at random, thus creating chaos and stops the heart from pumping and circulating blood. This would make the victim unconscious, collapse, and cease breathing.

Ventricular tachycardia or V-tach, on the other hand, occurs when the electrical system causes the ventricles to contract too quickly. Just like with V-fib, V-tach would make the patient unconscious, collapse, and cease breathing.

Both V-tach and V-fib can be corrected with an electric shock delivered by an AED. This portable electronic device will analyze the heart's rhythm and defibrillate or deliver an electric shock to help the heart's rhythm get back on track.

Using an AED

When a sudden cardiac arrest occurs, the first thing to do is notify the local emergency services immediately and commence CPR at once. CPR should be halted when an AED is available. CPR should only be paused when the defibrillation pads are ready. Several local guidelines instruct the use of an AED, which must be explicitly obeyed.

AED Precautions

The following are the general precautions that guide the use of an AED.

- Alcohol must not be used to clean the victim's chest. This is because alcohol is very flammable.

- Adult AEDs and pads must not be used on children below 8 years of age or individuals who weigh less than 55 pounds. It can only be used when there is no pediatric AED pad at hand.

- Similarly, pediatric AED pads should not be used on anyone over the age of 8 or those who weigh more than 55 pounds. This guideline is put in place because the pediatric pads are created to deliver lower energy meant specifically for children younger than 8 years or those who weigh below 55 pounds

- Do not touch the victim while the AED is in use and analyzing. Touching, moving, or displacing the victim might affect the analysis.

- Make sure no one is in contact with the victim before shocking the victim with an AED. No one should also be in contact with any of the resuscitation equipment.

- Touching the victim while defibrillating could shock you, so make sure no one is touching the victim before defibrillating.

- Remove the victim from flammable or combustible substances like gasoline or free-flowing oxygen before defibrillating. This is to prevent fire accidents.

- AEDs should not be used in a moving vehicle to ensure the authenticity of the results given.

- The victim must not be in any water while the responder is working on the AED.

- An AED cannot be used on a victim with a nitroglycerin patch or any other medical patch on the chest. Use a gloved hand to remove any patches on the chest before going ahead.

- There should be no use of mobile phones or radio within 6 feet of the AED. This is because radiofrequency interference (RFI), electromagnetic interference (EMI), and the infrared interference, which are all generated by the radio signals, can affect the analysis.

How to use an AED

There are different types of AEDs available, but they are all operated similarly, and their feature is quite similar to the electrode (defibrillation or AED) pads, the voice prompts, the visual displays, and the lighted buttons that guide responders on how to use an AED. The steps to use most AEDs are:

- Switch the AED on

- The bare chest of the victim should be wiped clean and dry with a small towel or a gauze pad to ensure the AED pads are accurately stuck on the chest.

- The AED pads should then be placed one after the other on the victim's chest.

- One pad should be placed on the upper right side of the chest while the other pad should be on the left chest.

- If necessary, plug the connector to the AED.

- Click on the 'analyst' button, which will prompt the AED to examine and determine the rhythms of the heart.

- Demand that all bystanders 'stand clear'. There should be no form of contact with the victim by anyone, while the AED is analyzing the heart rhythm. Any form of contact with the victim affects the AED analysis and produces a faulty reading.

- If the AED prompts that a shock is needed, then make sure, again, that no-one, yourself included, is touching the victim. Instruct everyone to stand clear.

- Push the 'shock' button to deliver the needed shock to reset the heart. Some AED models have a shock button which must be manually pushed to deliver the shock while other models deliver the shock automatically.

- If no shock is recommended or after the delivered shock, perform 5 cycles or 2 minutes of CPR. Continue to follow the instructions of the AED.

Once signs of life are seen, stop CPR, and monitor the victim's condition and breathing for any changes.

How to use an AED on Children and Infants

Compared to adults, children and infants hardly ever experience sudden cardiac arrests resulting from V-fib. The uncommon cases are usually because of traumatic accidents, airways and breathing problems, congenital heart disease, a hard blow to the chest, or sudden infant death syndrome. When a sudden cardiac arrest occurs, the first thing to do is make a call to the local emergency services.

AEDs with pediatric AED pads are designed to deliver lower levels of energy as is proper for children and infants under the age of 8 years or those who weigh less than 55 pounds. When available, make use of the pediatric-specific equipment. In cases when it is not available, you can use the AED designed for adults. Local protocols, as given by the medical director, and the manufacturer's instructions must be obeyed. The general steps and procedures guiding the use of AED on an adult are also observed here.

- First turn on the AED

- Expose the infant or child's chest and wipe it dry using a small towel or gauze pads

- The pediatric pads are then applied to the child's or infant's chest, one to the upper right and the other to the left side of the chest.

- It is important that the pads do not touch. To avoid that from happening, especially with infants or children with a small chest, one pad can be placed in the middle of the chest and the other pad placed at the back of the child or infant, right between the shoulder blades.

- When necessary, plug the connector to the AED.

- The AED will then analyze the heart rhythm of the child or infant either automatically or by pushing the 'analyze' button when prompted by the AED.

- All responders and bystanders are told to stand clear because touching the child or infant while analyzing can skewer the results.

- In cases when a shock is needed, make sure everyone, yourself included, is not touching the child. Instruct everyone to stand clear.

- Push the 'shock' button to deliver the necessary shock.

- If no shock is advised or after the necessary shock, perform 5 cycles or 2 minutes of CPR and continue to follow the instructions of the AED.

Once signs of life are observed, stop CPR, and monitor the victim's condition and breathing for any changes.

Special Situations

There are tricky or special situations sometimes that needs special attention while making use of the AED. Some of such situations include making use of the AED around water and on people with hypothermia, implantable devices, transdermal patches, trauma, jewelry, or body piercings. You might also get confuses if the protocols or AED instructions are different from what you are used to. It is best to understand situations like this can occur so that you can know what to do and respond appropriately.

AED around water

First, remove the victim from the water where he or she is in before defibrillating. Delivering a shock in water is dangerous to bystanders. Make sure there are no pools or bodies of water around the victim, the AED, or you. Remove all wet clothing to allow for proper attachment of the pads. Make sure the victim's chest is dry before attaching the AED pads.

In cases of rain, ensure to keep the victim as dry as possible and away from the rain. The victim's chest must be dried before the AED pads can be attached. While trying to create a dry environment, do not delay defibrillation. When all precautions are taken, and the manufacturer's instructions are followed, it is safe to use an AED, no matter the weather. Always avoid getting the AED or defibrillation pads wet.

Pacemakers and Implantable Cardioverter-Defibrillators

Individuals whose hearts beat too slowly beat too fast, skip beats, or whose hearts are weak often have a pacemaker implanted. These pacemakers are small, implantable devices that are often placed below the left collar bone, although they might be put somewhere. In place of pacemakers, some others have an ICD, implantable cardioverter-defibrillator, which is basically a mini AED. The ICDs immediately recognize the heart's irregular heartbeats and restore it to normal. Even with the pacemaker or an ICD, there are times the victim's heart beats irregularly.

When the implanted device is visible, or you become aware that the victim has one, the defibrillation pads must not be placed directly over the device. This is because the implanted device may interfere with the delivery of the shock to the heart. Simply adjust the AED pads placement and continue with the laid down instructions. In cases when you are not sure if the victim has had an AED implanted, the

AED can be used as needed. It will do no harm to the victim or the responder.

There is a possibility of a shock to the responder while performing CPR to a victim with implantable ICD when the ICD delivers a shock to the victim's heart. The risk of injury to the responders from the shock is minimal to none as the amount of electrical energy involved is minimal at best. Obey the precautions that are associated with ICDs, but there should be no hesitation in performing CPR and making use of the AED.

Transdermal Medication Patches
Some people receive medication through their skin, and this is called transdermal medication patches. A very common transdermal patch is the nitroglycerin patch that is used by those with a history of cardiac problems. A responder can absorb the medication through the skin, so gloves must be worn before defibrillation. There are other patches like nicotine patches that look like nitroglycerin patches. Do not waste time trying to recognize which is which. Just remove any patches that are on the victim's chest with a gloved hand and begin defibrillation. The AED electrode pads must never be placed directly on top of any medication patches.

Hypothermia
Hypothermia occurs when the body cannot keep warm. It is a life-threatening condition that causes the body to continually cool. There are several cases of successful resuscitation of victims even after prolonged exposure to cold. Responders must first begin with CPR

for victims that are not breathing before making use of an AED. The local protocols should be observed in situations like this.

For wet victims, remove any wet clothing and dry the chest before attaching the AED pads. Follow the instructions of the AED to indicate and deliver a shock. If the victim is still not breathing, then perform CPR and try to prevent further heat loss from the victim. Local protocols would dictate further shocks should be administered. Do not stop defibrillation or CPR while warming the victim. Unnecessary shaking of the victim with hypothermia can result in V-fib.

Chest Hair

There are occurrences when men with excessive chest hairs can interfere with the AED pads to skin connection. As time is of the essence, and these incidents rarely happen, make sure to attach the pads firmly to analyze the heart's rhythm as soon as possible. Press the pads firmly on the victim's chest to make sure they stay attached and not give a skewed reading.

If the AED is telling you to 'check pads' or a similar message, then remove the pads and replace them with other new ones. Some of the chest hairs can be pulled with the pad adhesive and solve the problem. Included in the AED kit should be spare defibrillation pads and a safety razor. Carefully shave the chest hair to avoid cuts and scrapes because they can interfere with the rhythm analysis.

Metal Surfaces

Delivering shock to a victim that is lying on metal surfaces like bleachers is safe as long as the proper safety measures are taken. Take care to note that the metal or conductive surface is not in contact with the defibrillation electrode pads. Also, make sure that no one is touching the victim, and everyone is standing clear before pressing the shock button.

Jewelry and Body Piercings

There is no need to remove the Jewelry and body piercings of the victim before using the AED. Their presence on the victim's body will do no harm. As time is of the essence, removing them from the body is reducing the chances of the victim to live. Take note, however, not to place the AED pads directly on the metallic jewelry or any body piercings on the victim. The AED pads placement can be adjusted if necessary.

Finally, it is one of the AED protocols to deliver three electric shocks and then perform CPR. This is not harmful, nor is it wrong, but new and improved methods based on scientific evidence allows for easy coordination of CPR and the AED. Simply make sure to obey the instructions of the AED device that is in use.

Trauma

AED can be used on victims who suffer from sudden cardiac arrest as a result of traumatic injuries. Defibrillation can be administered according to the local protocols.

Stroke

Stroke is the third leading cause of death and one of the leading causes of disability in the United States. It has been estimated that at least 800,000 Americans have a stroke in a year. Sometimes the effects of a stroke are permanent, and sometimes, the effects are reversible.

Just like all other illnesses, some signs warn that a stroke is about to happen. Sudden illness and strange sudden behavior are the common signs of an oncoming stroke or transient ischemic attack, also known as a mini-stroke. The signs specific to a stroke, however, include numbness or weakness of the arm, leg, or face. There is often visible facial drooping, and the victim often has trouble getting words out. Victims who suffer from strokes also often complain of a blinding and terrible headache, 'the worst one they have ever had.'

Victims suffering from stroke can easily be identified using the FAST technique. FAST stands for:

- **FACIAL DROOP:** One side of the victim's face will visibly droop. There would be numbness, weakness, or drooping on one side of the victim's face. It is often pronounced when the victim is asked to smile.

- **ARM WEAKNESS**: The victim also experiences weakness in one arm. Instruct the victim to lift both arms to their shoulder level for about 10seconds. The arm of a victim suffering from stroke would lower significantly from the other, and the arm would also rotate inwards.

- **SPEECH DIFFICULTY:** Victims suffering from a stoke will find it difficult to speak. The victim will also be unable to repeat simple sentences like 'the chicken crossed the road' or 'the sky is blue.'

- **TIME:** It is important to call for help immediately. Try to remember when the stroke began. Call the local emergency services for help right away.

It is only by paying attention to the signs of a stroke and reporting them immediately will go a long way in preventing any lasting damage to the brain. A mini-stroke is the clear warning of an impending stroke. The signs of stoke are not to be ignored even if they disappear after a couple of minutes or hours.

The best way to help a victim suffering from a stroke is to call for help immediately. Also, take note of the time the signs of stroke began. If the victim is unconscious, care for any life-threatening conditions and make sure the airway is open. If there is vomit or fluid in the person's mouth, position him or her on one side so the fluids drain out. Anything else in the mouth of an unconscious victim must be removed with a finger. Closely monitor the victim for any change in condition or breathing.

Check for non-life-threatening conditions in a conscious victim. A victim suffering from a stroke will likely be feeling anxious and afraid. Many times, the victim does not understand what is going on. Offer comfort and reassurances to the victim. Place the victim in a comfortable position and do not offer him or her anything to drink or eat.

First Aid Treatment during Breathing Emergencies

In cases when a child, an infant, or an adult is having trouble breathing, you can help the victim feel more comfortable by placing them in a comfortable position. Sitting is a more comfortable position than lying down because it is easier to breathe while sitting. If the victim is still conscious, remember to check for other injuries and conditions. Take note that the victim who is having trouble breathing would not find it easy to talk. If the victim is unable to speak, limit your questions to yes or no. Be sure to reassure the victim that everything would be okay to reduce the victim's anxiety. That might also help in making breathing easier. You can also glean information about the victim from the onlookers' present.

If the victim is hyperventilating due to emotions like excitement or fear, instruct the victim to breathe slowly and relax. Hyperventilation due to emotions may reduce to normal breathing if the victim is reassured and can calm down. If, after reassurance, the breathing does not slow down, the victim could have a serious medical problem.

An unconscious adult who is not breathing is likely suffering from a cardiac emergency. CPR with chest compressions is to begin immediately. If the adult victim is not breathing as a result of a respiratory cause like drowning or drug overdose, 2 rescue breaths are recommended after checking for breathing and before checking for severe bleeding. After that, CPR is to follow.

It is important to remember that for an individual who is not breathing, what he or she needs the most is oxygen. Without it, the brain, as well as other vital organs, begin to die. If the obstruction of air has gone on long enough, the victim loses consciousness, the heart stops beating, and the shutdown of the body systems soon follows.

For infants and children who are unconscious and unable to breathe, give 2 rescue breaths once you have checked for breathing status just before you scan for bleeding and begin CPR.

Choking

When an individual is choking, which happens to be a common enough breathing problem, the airway of such an individual is partially or completely blocked. A completely blocked airway is often because of a foreign object like food or a small toy, by swelling in the throat or mouth or by fluids. A partially blocked airway results in breathing with difficulty, the air getting in and out of the lungs results in coughs or wheezing sounds.

The signs of choking include:

- Either weak or forceful coughing.

- The clutching of the throat with one or both hands

- The inability to cough or speak or breathe or cry.

- High pitched noises while inhaling or breathing.

- Panic

- Loss of consciousness when blockage remains.

Choking Treatments

Several factors can cause an adult to choke, such as alcohol during and after meals, which dulls the nerves that aid swallowing, wearing dentures, swallowing poorly chewed food, eating while talking excitedly, playing, walking, or running with food or objects in the mouth and so on.

In infants and children, it is a very common cause of death, especially for those under the age of 5 because little children put about anything in their mouths especially small non-food items. However, food is what is most responsible for choking incidents among children. Food items that can cause choking in children include chewing gum, vitamins, grapes, hard candy, popcorn, and so on, while some of the non-food items that can cause choking in children include baby powder, coins, marbles, pen, marker caps, safety pins and so on.

If the victim is coughing forcefully, then allow the said victim to try to cough the object out. Anyone who has enough air to cough and to speak has enough air to breathe. You should encourage the person to keep breathing. When it is seen that a victim has breathing problems or is choking, the local emergency services must be notified at once.

There are several ways of removing the object that is lodged in the airway of a conscious victim with a blocked airway. 5 back blows, which is immediately followed by 5 abdominal thrusts, is a highly effective way of clearing the obstruction to the airway. Place yourself slightly behind the victim to deliver the back blows correctly. Put one hand diagonally across the chest to offer support and bend the victim forward at the waist so that the upper airway is parallel to the ground. Then firmly hit the victim between the shoulder blades with the heel of the freehand.

Delivering abdominal thrusts requires you to stand or kneel at the back of the victim. Your arms should be wrapped around the person's waist and, with a finger or two of one hand, locate the navel. The other hand should be rolled into a fist with the thumb side sticking against the victim's abdomen. The fisted hand should then deliver quick, upward thrusts into the abdomen.

Each of the back blow and the abdominal thrusts is a different and separate effort to remove the obstruction. 5 sets of back blows and five abdominal thrusts are done repeatedly until the object is removed or the person becomes unconscious. A conscious child needs less force during back blows and abdominal thrusts.

Anyone who choked and had been given abdominal thrusts, back blows, and/or chest thrusts for a clear airway needs medical attention to clear out any internal injuries or damages to the airway.

Some special conditions need a little finessing when trying to help. To help a large person or heavily pregnant woman, it is often impossible to reach around people in this category. Chest thrusts should be given to them instead. For a conscious adult, a chest thrust is like an abdominal thrust, the only difference being the hand placement. Chest thrusts need you to place your fists against the center of the victim's backbone. You then grab your fist with the other hand and thrust quickly into the chest.

If you happen to find yourself choking when you are alone, you can still help yourself by bending over and pressing your abdomen against a firm object like a railing, the back of a chair, or a kitchen sink. Be careful not to bend over objects with a sharp edge or ones with corners because they might hurt you. In the same vein, exercise caution while leaning over elevated rails. You can also give yourself abdominal thrusts as you would administer to another person. Abdominal thrusts can also help a choking victim in a wheelchair.

A conscious infant who cannot cough, cry or breathe needs a combination of 5 back blows accompanied by 5 chest thrusts. The back blows are administered when the infant is properly positioned on the forearm. One hand and forearm are placed on the child's back, cradling the back of the head and the other hand and forearm on the front of the infant. With the thumb and fingers, hold the infant's jaw as the infant is sandwiched between your forearms.

Place the infant in a face-down position along your forearm. Place said forearm on your thigh to provide adequate support. The positioning on the thigh also ensures that the head of the infant is lower than the chest. The head of the infant must be supported by clasping the jaw between the forefinger and the thumb. Hit the infant between the shoulder blades in 5 firms back blows. Each of the back blows is an intentional and isolated venture to remove the obstructing object.

To give chest thrusts, the infant must be in a face-up position. This is done by placing a hand and forearm on the child's back supporting the back of the head and the other hand and forearm on the child's front. With the thumb and forearm, hold the infant's jaw while the infant is firmly sandwiched between the forearms.

The arm supporting the infant's back must be lowered onto the opposite thigh. The head of the infant should be lower than the chest to help in dislodging the object. The pads of two or three fingers should be placed at the center of the infant's chest towards the feet and just below the nipple line. The pads of the fingers will compress the breastbone. Compression should be about 5 times at about an inch and a half before allowing the breastbone to return to its normal position. Remember to keep the fingers in close contact with the breastbone.

The sets of 5 back blows and 5 chest thrusts must be continually administered until the dislodged object is expelled; the infant can cough, cry or breathe on his or her own, or the infant loses consciousness. Back blows and chest thrusts can be given effectively while sitting, standing, or kneeling just as long as the infant's head is lower than the chest, and your thigh supports the infant. It is safer to sit if the infant's head is too big or your hands are too small. The force applied during back blows and chest thrusts must be less than that applied to an adult or even a child. This is because the excessive application of force can lead to internal injuries. An unconscious child must be placed on a firm, flat surface, and CPR takes place immediately beginning with compressions.

First Aid Treatment for Environmental Emergencies

There are two types of environmental emergencies, which are heat-related illnesses and cold-related emergencies. Exposure to extreme heat or cold can cause serious effects on a person. Here are some ways to help prevent the deterioration of the illnesses and emergencies before the EMS personnel arrive.

Heat-Related Illnesses

Heat cramps, the least severe of the unholy trio of heat-related illnesses, are still very painful muscle spasms that often occur in the abdomen and legs. They are the warning signs of worse things to come. Moving the victim to a cool place to rest will go a long way in caring for heat cramps. Fluid having electrolytes and carbohydrates like a commercial sports drink, milk, or fruit juice should be given to the victim as well. Water can also do the trick. Stretch the muscle lightly and gently massage the area. Salt tablets will only worsen the situation and should not be taken. The victim can resume activities when the cramps stop, and there are no further signs of illnesses. The victim should, however, continue taking plenty of fluids. A close eye also needs to be kept on the victim for further signs of heat-related illnesses.

Heat exhaustion, the more severe condition, shows symptoms like flushed or cool skin, nausea, dizziness, exhaustion, or weakness. When noticed early, heat exhaustion is reversible. The victim must first be taken out of the heat into a cool area with circulating air. Clothing should be removed or loosened. Cool, wet cloths like towels should be applied. Make sure the clothes are always wet. Fanning or spraying the victim with water also helps. If the victim can swallow, then offer him or her small amounts of cool fluid-like fruit juice or a commercial sports drink. The victim should take about 4 ounces of fluid every fifteen minutes. The victim should still be in a comfortable position and be closely observed for changes in condition. The victim cannot resume normal activities for the rest of the day.

If there is no change in the victim's condition, they cannot take fluids, they vomit, or there is a noticeable change in consciousness, reach out to the local emergency services because they are indications that the victim's condition is worsening. Stop administering fluids and lay the victim on his or her side to make sure the airway stays open. Continue to observe for any changes in breathing.

Heatstroke is the deadliest of heat-related illnesses. When there are signs of heatstroke, the preferred method of helping before the local emergency services arrive is to cool the body of the victim quickly. That can be done by plunging the victim into the cool water from the neck down. If that is not possible, then spray the victim with water. The victim should also be washed with towels that have been dipped in ice-cold water. The towels should be dipped intermittently. The victim can be covered with bags of ice as another alternative. If there is no way to measure the victim's temperature accurately, then apply the rapid cooling methods for as long as 20 minutes or until there is a physical improvement in the victim's condition.

Cold-Related Emergencies

The two types of cold-related emergencies are frostbite and hypothermia. Frostbite, which occurs when body parts are exposed to cold, shows its signs in waxy skin, lack of feeling in the affected area, and swelling. Blisters occur in serious cases of frostbite. The first thing to do in cases of frostbite is to call for help from the local emergency services. Until help arrives, handle the frostbitten area with care. Gently remove the wet clothing and jewelry from the affected area if it is possible. Do not rub the affected area because that would cause further damage to the soft tissues. If there is a chance that the affected area will refreeze, help will soon arrive, or you are close to a medical facility, then don't try to rewarm the frostbitten area. Minor frostbites can be rapidly rewarmed by skin-to-skin contact like a warm hand.

The more serious frostbite injuries need gentle soaking in water that is no warmer than about 105°F. When there is no thermometer, you can test the water yourself by touch. If the water is at an uncomfortable temperature, then it is too warm to your touch. Allow the frostbitten area to stay in the water until the normal color is restored, and the area feels warm again. Ensure to bandage the area loosely with a dry sterile dressing. Frostbitten fingers and toes can be bandaged with cotton or gauze between them. Do well not to break any blisters. Take measures to prevent the onset of hypothermia. Closely monitor the condition of the victim. While caring for frostbite victims, do not administer ibuprofen or any other type of anti-inflammatory drugs (NSAIDs).

Victims who suffer from hypothermia are unable to keep their body warm. As a result, the entire body cools, and unless immediate care is given, the victim is liable to die. Several circumstances lead to hypothermia, and that includes the ingestion of substances like alcohol, certain drugs, or medication that interfere with the ability of the body to control the core temperature. There are also certain medical conditions like diabetes or cardiovascular diseases that interfere with the body's ability to regulate body temperature. Extended exposure to cold conditions, as well as wet clothing, can also lead to hypothermia. Local emergency services should be notified at once the signs of hypothermia like shivering, numbness, indifference, loss of consciousness, and a glassy stare presents itself.

Until the EMS personnel arrive, try making the victim comfortable. Gently prod the victim to a warm place. Take off the wet clothing and dry off the victim. Give the victim dry clothes to put on. Gradually warm up the body by wrapping the victim up in blankets and plastic sheeting. The blankets and plastic sheeting hold in the body heat and allow the body to warm itself up gradually. Ensure the head is also covered to hold the body heat in.

If help is far off, carefully place the victim near a heat source. Heat pads or heat sources, like containers filled with warm water, can also be applied to the victim. Do not place the victim directly near the heat source. Ensure there is a barrier like a towel or blanket between the heat source and the victim. Carefully observe the victim ensure the heat source does not burn the victim. Give warm fluids to conscious and alert victims. Do not offer alcohol or caffeine to the victim. This is because alcohol can lead to heat loss, and caffeine leads to dehydration. Closely monitor the breathing and condition of the victim for any changes as well as signs of shock.

The victim may be unconscious in cases of severe hypothermia. The victim's breathing may have also stopped or slowed. Due to the rigidity of the muscles, the body will feel stiff. Check for the breathing of no more than 10 seconds. If the victim is not breathing, then perform immediate CPR. Until the emergency medical services (EMS) personnel arrive, continue to warm the victim. If an AED, automated external defibrillator, is available, be prepared to make use of it.

First Aid Treatment for Head Injuries

Trauma is the most common cause of injuries to the brain and the spinal cord. Injuries to the head are to be treated with extreme caution and swift action because it can lead to the death or deterioration of the health of the victim. Call the local emergency services immediately; there is a victim with brain injuries.

Treatment for Skull Fractures

- INSPECT THE VICTIM'S SKULL: The first thing to do is to check for bleeding. If the victim is not bleeding, then inspect the skull for any depressed fractures. If the victim is bleeding is minor, first stop the bleeding by applying even and firm pressure to the bleeding site with a piece of clean cloth or a piece of gauze. The direct pressure applied will slow down the bleeding and allow for clotting. Inspect the skull for signs of depression, irregular shape, and compound fractures then gently palpate the victim's skull. The presence of pain, tenderness, or swelling indicates the possibility of a fracture.

- CONSIDER IRRIGATION: If you believe the victim does not have an open fracture, then you may go ahead to clean the wound. However, if you suspect that the victim might have an open fracture, cleaning or irrigating the wounds means introducing bacteria into the meninges or the brain. The presence of bacteria in the brain increases the chances of permanent damages. Stop the bleeding and wait for the EMS personnel.

- CHECK FOR SIGNS OF CRANIAL TRAUMA: The skull should be inspected for signs of basilar skull fracture. A break in any of the bones at the base of the skull leads to a basilar skull fracture. A basilar skull fracture is evident when there are bruising around the eyes or 'raccoon eyes,' as they are otherwise called, there is bruising behind the ears, and there is blood in the eardrum. A tear in the dura mater of the victim can lead to the leaking of the CSF. Symptoms that signify a CSF leak are just like the symptoms of other brain injuries. CSF leaks can lead to the clear drainage of the nose of the ears. There have also been reports by victims of a sweet and salty taste in their mouths. A lot of CSF leaks occur with basilar fractures. Ear bleeding is another indication of cranial trauma. Victims with suspected CSF leaks or visible ear bleeds need medical attention immediately.

- ALLOW DRAINAGE: In cases of CSF leakage or bleeding from the ears or nose, don't try to control the drainage or bleeding. Attempting to control the bleeding or the drainage can lead to an increase in the intracranial pressure (ICP). An increase in the ICP can cause further damage to the brain. Victims should be discouraged from coughing, sneezing, or any other activity that increases the pressure in the head.

- SIT UPRIGHT: Make sure the victim remains sitting in an upright position. This is because lying down can increase ICP and further complicate the injuries.

- MONITOR VITAL SIGNS: While waiting for the local emergency services, closely monitor the victim's condition, consciousness, and breathing.

Treatment for Scalp Injuries

There are a good number of arteries and veins all passing through the scalp to their various destinations. Due to the structure of tissues, the damaged blood vessels in the scalp are unable to contrast. That means a cut in the scalp will lead to profuse bleeding or severe bruising. The loss of a significant amount of blood can lead to shock for the victim. Treating wounds in the scalp is similar to treating open wounds in other parts of the body. However, the responder should be careful because of any underlying fracture. There might also be traumatic brain injuries associated with scalp injuries.

- STOP THE BLEEDING: This is the first step in treatment for victims with scalp injuries. For victims with a suspected skull fracture, do not apply direct pressure to the injury. Simply cover the wound with gauze instead.

- CONSIDER IRRIGATION: Scalp injuries with open fractures should not be irrigated or cleaned. This is to avoid the introduction of bacteria to the brain. Irrigate the wound only if you are absolutely sure there is no open fracture in the skull.

- DRESS THE WOUND: Place gauze over the wound and apply firm pressure to stop the bleeding. A gauze roll or elastic net dressing can be used to keep the gauze in place.

- CONSIDER SHOCK: The victim could go into shock depending on how much blood is lost. Keep an eye on the victim for chock while waiting for the EMS personnel.

Treatment for Traumatic Brain Injury

There are several types of brain injuries. The rain injuries from birth or congenital brain injuries and acquired brain injuries. Brain injuries can be acquired from either a traumatic event caused by an external mechanical force like an accident, or a non-traumatic event, like a stroke or an infection. In the event of a traumatic brain injury, time is of the essence. It is important to call the local emergency services immediately. While waiting for help to arrive, here are a few things that can be down to make the victim more comfortable.

- CONSIDER PERSONAL AND VICTIM SAFETY: If the victim is antagonistic, then let him or her be. Give the victim the needed space and encourage the bystanders to step back. It is possible the victim is confused, and further antagonizing the patient is worsening the victim's condition.

- MONITOR THE VICTIM: The victims who show signs of traumatic brain injury are encouraged to sit and relax while their condition is monitored closely. The mental status of the victim is evaluated through casual conversation. Basic questions are asked about the date and location to prove orientation. The casual conversation offers some ideas as to the mental status of the victim. Check the pupils and take note of the respiration rate, the blood pressure, and the heart rate of the victim to set up a baseline for further comparison.

- CONSIDER IMMOBILIZATION: Traumatic brain injuries can be associated with spinal injuries. In the interest of preventing further complications, the victim should stay immobile in the same position as the accident, if possible, to prevent spinal injuries.

First Aid for Allergies

An allergy is the response of our body to foreign substances called allergens. Common allergens include pollen dust, animal dander, drugs, and food substances. An allergic reaction happens when the defense system of the body reacts to substances that are foreign to the body, though those substances might not be harmful.

The body produces a chemical called histamine, which causes allergic symptoms such as swelling, sneezing, coughing, and difficulty breathing.

Allergic reactions depend on what the body reacts to. Parts of the body that react are the airways, nose, mouth, digestive system and skin

A severe allergic reaction is called anaphylaxis. It could result in shock, a drop in blood pressure, or difficulty breathing. It can also lead to cardiac arrest or respiratory failure.

Symptoms of an allergic reaction

- Red, itchy rash

- Vomiting

- Diarrhea

- Itching

- Sneezing

- Red, itchy, watery eyes

- Swollen hands, feet or face

- Difficulty breathing

- Swelling of the tongue

- Confusion

- Dizziness

First aid for allergies

For mild allergies:

- Administer antihistamines for red and itchy skin. Antihistamine blocks the histamine receptors, which prevent symptoms of allergic reactions.

- Topical creams that contain corticosteroids can be applied for swelling and itching of the skin

- Administer decongestants for nasal congestion. They help clear the nose.

- Administer eye drops for itchy eyes.

For skin allergies:

- Clean the area with soap and water for at least 10 minutes

- Victim should take a cool bath

- Apply anti-itching lotion such as calamine for at least three to four times to relieve itching

- Massage swollen areas with 1% hydrocortisone creams

- Victim should wash clothing and footwear in hot water

For insect stings:

- Remove the insect with a straight-edged object. Avoid squeezing the insect as it might release more venom into the skin

- Clean the area with soap and water.

- Use an antiseptic after washing the affected area

- Apply anti-itching lotion or hydrocortisone cream

- Apply a cold compress to swollen areas

- Cover the area with a clean bandage

- Administer an antihistamine to reduce swelling and itching

- Administer pain relieve drugs

Call the local emergency services if the victim is:

- Experiencing difficulty breathing.

- Complaining of tightening throats.

- Prone to severe allergic reactions

- Unconscious.

Anaphylaxis

This is a severe allergic reaction that occurs after exposure to allergens and could lead to loss of consciousness, respiratory failure, or cardiac arrest. It occurs when the body responds to an allergen suddenly and goes into shock.

Symptoms of anaphylaxis:

- Itchy skin

- Nausea

- Vomiting

- Diarrhea

- Troubled breathing

- Swelling of the body parts

- Dizziness

- Anxiety

- Weak and fast pulse

- Low blood pressure

- Heart attack

- First aid for anaphylaxis

- Check if the victim has an emergency adrenaline injection

- Administer the adrenaline injection

- Doses of adrenaline can be administered at five-minute intervals

- Keep the victim calm

- Help the victim lay on their back

- Keep the victim comfortable

- Cover the victim with a blanket

- Turn the victim on their side if they're bleeding or vomiting

- Ensure that the clothing on the victim are loose to allow breathing

- Observe the breathing of the victim

- In case there are no signs of breathing or movement, do CPR - about 100 chest presses per minute

Precautions
- Do not administer any oral medication or lift the head of the victim

First Aid Treatment for Burns

A burn is damage to tissues of the skin from contact with fire, hot fluids or objects, chemicals, electric current, or radiation.

The location of the burn must be considered. For burns that affect the face, nose, mouth, or neck, there is a tendency that there will be an injury in the airways, which will cause swelling to block the airways and trouble breathing.

If the burns are on the chest, the affected tissues may not allow movement of the chest wall. This will prevent adequate breathing.

Burns on the arms, legs, fingers, or toes might tighten the blood vessels and prevent blood flow, which might affect the function of the limbs later.

To figure out how to treat a burn, one must decide whether the burn is a minor or a major one.

What is a Major Burn?

Major burns are classified as a second degree and third-degree burns. They are burns that affect and damage part or all layers of the skin resulting in dry and leathery skin. The nerve endings of the affected areas also suffer great damage. The tissues of areas with major burns are black, brown, or while with little to no blisters. For the most part, the burns like that are larger than three inches, and they are around delicate parts of the body like the face, the hands, the buttocks, the groin, the feet, or a major joint.

Treatment for Major Burns

- Move the victim from the source of the burn.

- Remove any burning material from the victim. Do not remove any clothing stuck to the skin.

- Remove any tightly fitted item from the body of the victim, such as rings, jewelry, and belts.

- Cover the affected area loosely with a moist, clean cloth or bandage.

- Separate the fingers and toes with dry, clean nonstick bandages.

- Raise the affected area above the heart level.

- Cover the victim with a blanket

- In case of a facial burn, have the victim sit up.

- Observe the pulse and breath of the victim to check for shock

- Call for medical aid

Precautions
- Do not put the affected area in water.

- Do not apply any ointments, butter, ice, spray, or cream

- Do not infect the affected area with germs by breathing or coughing on it

- Do not give the victim anything to ingest

- In case of airway burn, do not put a pillow beneath the head of the victim, it might block the airways.

What is a Minor Burn?

First degree burns are classified as minor burns as well as second degree covering only a small area of the body, less than three inches. The surface of the skin is usually red with blisters and do cause an amount of pain.

First Aid for Minor Burns

- Remove the source of the burn

- Cool the burn by running the affected area under cool water

- Remove any tightly fitted items such as rings, belts from the affected area.

- If blisters break, clean the area and apply an antibiotic ointment gently.

- Cover the affected area with clean, nonstick bandage or cloth

- Apply a petroleum-based ointment two to three times a day

- Administer pain relief drugs such as acetaminophen or ibuprofen

Precautions

- Do not break blisters. The blisters are holding fluid to protect the affected area from infection.

- Do not apply butter, oil, lotions, or cream.

Electrical Burns

Electrical burns may be caused by sources of electricity such as sun, lightning, or contact with household current. Sometimes the effects of electrical injuries may not be obvious initially, because the entrance and exit of the electric current may not be identified.

The electrical currents move towards the nerves and muscles, and they become damaged. When muscle damage occurs, there is a break-down of the muscle fibers and release of chemicals, which cause an imbalance in the body's electrolytes and could lead to kidney damage.

First Aid for Electrical Burns

- Remove the source of the electricity with a dry, nonconductor such as wood or plastic

- Cover the victim with warm clothing to prevent being chilled

- Cover the affected area with a clean, nonstick cloth or bandage.

Precautions

- Do not touch the victim is still in contact with the source of electricity

- Do not move the victim unless in immediate danger

Chemical Burns

Chemical burns are caused by chemical substances such as strong acids, bases, paint thinner, and fuel. The chemicals, when in contact with the skin, creates heat. The Effects of mild chemicals may not be felt at first until a few hours later, when the affected area becomes red and causes pain.

First Aid for Chemical Burns

- Remove the source of the burn.

- Place the affected area under running cool water for at least ten minutes to flush off the chemical.

- If the chemical is a dry substance, remove the remaining substance with a brush before flushing the affected area.

- Remove any material or clothing that had contact with the chemical

- Cover the affected area loosely with a clean, nonstick bandage or cloth.

- In case of any continuous burning sensation, flush the affected area with running cool water again

First Aid for Concussions

The mild traumatic injury to the brain is also known as a concussion. It results in a sudden short loss of brain function. It can occur as a result of a blow to the head, the violent and continuous shaking of the head in a back and forth motion, during falls or car accidents. Among the several effects of a concussion are headaches, concentration problems, poor memory, imbalance, and coordination problems. The appearance of the effects varies, sometimes appearing immediately, sometimes not showing for hours or even days.

A concussion is caused by a violent blow to the head, neck, or upper body. Causes of concussion include falls, vehicle accidents, or collision during sports activities.

Symptoms of concussion include

- Headache

- Blurry vision

- Confusion

- Dizziness

- Fatigue

- Ringing in the head

- Irritability

- Nausea

- Vomiting

- Sleep disturbance

- Sensitivity to light and noise

- Loss of consciousness

- Brief loss of memory

First aid for concussions

- Lay the victim still on the floor.

- Keep the victim's head and shoulders higher than the rest of the body.

- Try to stop any bleeding by applying pressure on the injured area with a clean cloth

- Apply a cold compress to the injury such as a piece of ice wrapped in a towel to reduce swelling

- Administer paracetamol to relieve the pain

- Observe for changes in the alertness and breathing of the patient

- Allow the victim to rest adequately

Precautions

- Do not move the victim unless necessary

- Do not remove any clothing from the victim

- Do not apply pressure if the bleeding is from the head

- Do not administer non-steroidal anti-inflammatory drugs (NSAIDs) such as aspirin or ibuprofen as they can cause bleeding

- Do not allow the victim to take alcohol or take part in any strenuous activity

First Aid treatment for Asthma

Asthma is a condition in which the tube that carries air to your lungs become swollen and narrow. It is a disease that obstructs the flow of air to the lungs. The airways to the lungs become swollen and get filled up with mucus. This makes it difficult to breathe. It can also trigger coughing and a whistling sound when breathing.

Asthma is non-communicable. It cannot be transferred by contact from anyone suffering from the disease.

What is an Asthma Attack?

An asthma attack is the worsening of asthma symptoms. This happens suddenly and, most times, caused by exposure to triggers that should be avoided.

When an asthma attack occurs, the airways of the lungs become really swollen and produce extra mucus. The mucus is thicker and blocks the airways. The muscles of the airway also tighten, and this makes breathing difficult.

During an attack, one experiences shortness of breath and difficulty breathing. There is also whistling (wheezing) sound produced when breathing in and out and coughing.

It is possible to go for a long period without having asthma attacks, but there could be worsened symptoms when exposed to asthma triggers such as exposure to dust or cold air.

Causes of Asthma Attack

The immune system of asthma patients is usually oversensitive. This makes them develop an asthma attack when exposed to triggers. A trigger is anything that irritates the airway. Common triggers include:

- Dust mites

- Pollens

- Molds

- Cockroach wastes

- Pet dander

- Air pollutants

- Smoke

- Exercise

- Intense emotions

- Upper respiratory infections

- Gastroesophageal reflux disease (GERD)

- Cold air

- Stress

Symptoms of Asthma Attack

The severity of asthma attacks is determined by how severe the symptoms are and might interfere with one's daily activities. Mild asthma attacks often occur for asthma patients, and the symptoms usually go away after a few hours of treatment, but severe asthma symptoms need immediate medical attention.

There are early warning signs that occur before an asthma attack. By recognizing these signs, one can prevent an asthma attack or reduce its severity.

Early Signs of an Asthma Attack

- Weakness when exercising

- Wheezing or coughing after an exercise

- Frequent coughing, especially during the night

- Shortness of breath

- Reduced peak flow meter readings

- Trouble sleeping

- Feeling of tiredness or moodiness

- Signs of cold allergies such as the runny nose, sneezing, sore throat, nasal congestion, etc.

Management of these early symptoms with treatment as soon as they are recognized helps prevent severe cases of asthma attacks.

Symptoms of an asthma attack include:

- Rapid breathing

- Severe wheezing when breathing in and out

- Non-stop coughing

- Chest tightness

- Retractions - tightened neck and chest muscles

- Difficulty talking

- Anxiety

- Paleness

- Sweating

- Blue lips and fingernails

Risk Factors for Asthma Attack

Everyone who has asthma has the risk of having an asthma attack. There are increased risks if you've:

i. Had a severe asthma attack in the past

ii. Been previously admitted or taken to the emergency room for asthma

iii. Been intubated for asthma attack before

iv. Used more than two rescue inhalers in a month

v. Have a chronic health condition such as cardiovascular or chronic lung diseases, or sinusitis.

Complications of Asthma Attack

Asthma attacks could interrupt your daily activities such as sleep, work, school, and exercise and of those who live around you. It makes you visit the emergency room often and could be stressful and expensive. In severe cases, it could lead to respiratory arrest and death.

First Aid for Asthma Attack

1. Sit the individual uprightly and loosen any tight clothing. Be calm and reassuring.

2. Assist such individual to use prescribed asthma medication such as an inhaler

3. If there's no prescribed medication or such medication is absent, use a rescue inhaler from a first aid kit. Avoid using any other person's inhaler since you cannot be sure the medication is right for you. Also, it isn't sanitary and you risk transferring infection.

To use the inhaler with spacer:

i. Remove the cap and shake the inhaler well.

ii. Insert inhaler into the spacer.

iii. Make the patient breathe out completely and then insert the spacer mouthpiece firmly into the mouth of the patient.

iv. Press the inhaler once to give a puff

v. Make the patient breathe in slowly through the mouth and hold the breath for about ten seconds

vi. Give the patient four puffs, waiting for about one minute before giving the next puff.

vii. After four puffs, wait for four minutes to see if there's still troubled breathing. If yes, give another four puffs.

viii. If there is little or no improvement after these, give four to eight puffs every twenty minutes until an ambulance arrives or professional medical care is given.

To use an inhaler without a spacer:

i. Remove the cap and shake the inhaler well.

ii. Make the patient breathes out away from the inhaler.

iii. Insert the inhaler mouthpiece firmly into the mouth of the patient.

iv. Press the inhaler once as the patient breaths in slowly and deeply and remove the inhaler.

v. Make the patient hold the breath for about four seconds and then breathe out slowly.

vi. Give four puffs. Remember to shake the inhaler before each puff.

Note:

Do not assume drowsiness is a sign of improvement. It could be that asthma is worsening.

Do not assume improvement if you do not hear wheezing. The lungs could be so tight that there is not enough air movement to make the wheezing sound. It is called 'silent chest.' It could mean that asthma is worsening.

In case of a severe allergic reaction, administer adrenaline autoinjector (Epi-pen) before using asthma relief medication.

First Aid for Tendons and Fractures

The body is made up of bones and muscles. The bones make up the skeleton, and the muscles make up the flesh. The bones and the muscles are all connected by the tendons and ligaments that provide the needed support, shape, and stability to the body. The muscles are the soft tissues of the body. Many of the more than 600 muscles are attached to the bones by the aid of the tendons. The muscles move when electrical impulses from the brain go down to the muscles via the nerves, causing it to contract or relax as necessary. The loss of nerve control to a muscle is called paralysis. When that happens, the nearby muscle takes over.

The 200 bones of the body form the skeleton, which protects the internal organs of the body. The bones are strong and dense and do not injure easily, but when they do, they are often painful. As the years go by, the bones weaken. This is what causes older people to become more susceptible to bone injuries because they have brittle bones. Osteoporosis is the term for the gradual weakening of the bones. The joint is the connecting point for two or more bones and the ligaments hold the bones together at their connecting spot.

The types of injuries common to the muscles, the bones, and the joints are:

- Fractures

- Dislocations

- Sprains

- Strains

Fractures

A fracture occurs when there is a complete break, a chip, or a crack in a bone. There are times when even a twisting movement, a blow, or a fall leads to a fracture. Fractures can either be open or closed. An open wound is often involved with an open fracture. Open fractures occur when the end of bone tears through the skin. When an object breaks the skin and into the bone, like a bullet, it also causes an open fracture. The skin is not broken in a closed fracture. While a closed fracture is more common, an open fracture is riskier. This is because open fractures come with the risk of infection and severe bleeding. Fractures are usually only life-threatening if large bones are involved, if it severs an artery or if it affects breathing. Since a fracture is not always obvious, the cause of injury indicates as to if a victim has a fracture. Falling off a significant height or a car crash can lead to a fracture.

Dislocation

Dislocations are often more evident than fractures. A dislocation occurs when a bone at a joint moves away from its normal position. The movement comes with a show of force, often occurring as a result of a great or violent force pushing at the ligaments that hold the bones together. The function of a joint is invalidated when a bone moves out of place. A hollow end, bump, or a ridge then forms when none ought to be.

Sprains

The tearing of the ligaments from the joint is called a sprain. Even though mild sprains swell, they often heal quickly. That said, ignoring the signs of a sprain, and becoming too active too soon leads to the reactivation of the sprain, causing further pain and weakness of the joint and leading to a more severe sprain. A severe sprain can occur alongside a fracture or dislocation at the joint. The joints most susceptible to sprains are the joints of the ankle, the knee, the fingers, and the wrist.

Strains

When the tendons or muscles are stretched and torn, it is said to be a sprain. Strains occur when the muscle is overworked or by attempting to lift something heavy. Strains often occur in the muscles of the back, the thigh, the neck, or that of the lower back.

In any of the four common injuries, severe cases are often accompanied by:

- A great deal of pain. The affected areas become very painful to touch and move

- The affected area becomes significant swelling and bruising.

- The affected area would be deformed, twisted, or bent unnaturally. There might also be the presence of abnormal lumps, ridges, and hollows.

- The affected area cannot function properly.

- There would be bone fragments sticking out of the wound.

- The victim may hear or feel a pop or a snap as at the time of injury

- The victim may also feel the bones grating at the site of injury

- The affected areas become numb, cold, and tingly.

- The cause of injury might indicate the severity of the injury.

- The local emergency services should be noticed if

- The deformity is obvious.

- There is discoloration as well as moderate or severe swelling

- A snap or a pop was felt and/or heard as at the time of injury

- There is a bone sticking out of the injured site

- There is an open wound with a fracture

- The affected part cannot be used normally

- The injured part is numb and cold

- The injury occurred around the neck, the head, or the spine.

- The victim is having trouble breathing

- The injury cause is severe

Until the emergency medical personnel arrive, any injuries to the muscle, bone, and joints can be taken care of using the RICE mnemonic.

REST: Be careful not to move or straighten the affected area

IMMOBILIZE: Make sure to keep the injured area steady in the position it was found. Only the injured area should be splinted if the victim is to be moved or taken to the nearest medical facility. Reducing movement to the injured area prevents further damage.

COLD: Apply ice or cold water to the affected area for about 20 minutes. Put a barrier, a thin one, between the bare skin and the ice. If the victim cannot stand icing for 20 minutes, then ice the injured area for periods of 10 minutes. It is important to ice the affected area because icing reduces the pain, any swelling, and also reduces any internal bleeding. There has been no evidence to prove that the application of heat is beneficial to any muscle, bone, and joint injury.

ELEVATE: Elevate or raise the affected area only when it does not cause or worsen the pain. The elevation of the affected area helps to reduce the swelling.

Splinting An Injury

One of the best ways of preventing further injury is to splint the injured part. This will lead to the restriction of movement and is best done if the victim is to be moved to a hospital. If the act of splinting causes more pain to the victim, then it is better not to splint at all. The splint must also be positioned where the injury is found. For fractures, the joints above and below the injury site must be splinted. The same principle applies to the bones of sprains as well as joint injuries.

Splinting materials must be soft and padded to ensure the comfort of the victim. Proper circulation should be checked before and after splinting to make sure that the splint is not secured too tight. The various methods of splinting include

- **Anatomic splints** which make use of the victim's body. For instance, an injured leg can be bound to an uninjured leg.

- **Soft splints** which bind the injured area to soft materials like a folded blanket or towel or pillow or a folded triangular bandage. A sling is a type of soft bandage.

- **Rigid splints** make use of materials like padded boards, newspapers, or padded metal strips to bind to the injured site.

- The ground can serve as support for the affected area.

Once the injury is splinted, continue the application of ice to the affected area. Be sure to keep the victim for getting cold or overheated and continue to offer reassurances.

Chapter 5

Prevention and Preparedness: How to Stop Injuries from Happening

Injuries are costly. They have led to the disability and death of thousands of people in the United States alone every year. In 2007, about 124,000 Americans died from the injuries sustained. The unintentional injuries were the leading cause of death in that year among persons between 1 to 44 years of age. Motor crashes took the leading cause of death, closely followed by poisoning and falls. In that same year, 2007, approximately 34.3 million Americans sustained nonfatal injuries but still needed medical attention.

These unintentional injuries result in the loss of billions of dollars in forms of lost wages, medical expenses, property damage, insurance, and several other indirect costs. While injuries are not always inevitable, being prepared and having full knowledge of the safety procedures can help reduce the risk, prevent the further deterioration of injuries, and save the lives of the victims involved.

Several factors affect the risk of an individual getting injured. Among those factors are age, gender, economic status, geographical location, alcohol misuse, and abuse. Individuals under the age of 39 have the highest number of nonfatal injuries while people who are aged 40 and above recorded a high number of death from injuries sustained. Men are more likely to sustain injuries than women. They are also twice as likely to die from their injuries or sustain a fatal injury than women. The environment and economic status of people also affect the possibility of suffering from injuries, whether fatal or non-fatal. People in rural areas are more likely to sustain injuries than those in a metropolitan area. Also, injuries are more likely in low-income areas than high-income ones. Alcohol misuse and abuse is a common cause of injuries among teenagers and adults. In 2008, it was recorded that 32 percent of all the car deaths were alcohol-related. A huge number of people who die due to falls, drowning, and fires are also reported to be under the influence of alcohol.

While statistics show that injuries are more common to individuals of certain age and gender, the injuries themselves have more to do with behavior than age or gender. A lot of the injuries sustained are preventable but occur due to the way the victims interacted with the potential dangers around them. The risk of an injury can be prevented by taking the following steps.

- Understand the risk involved

- Take the needed measures in the right direction. By changing certain behaviors, the risk of injuries to yourself and those around you reduce drastically.

- Be alert to your environment and think safely. Avoid potentially harmful conditions as well as activities that increase the risk of injuries.

- Take the necessary precautions, like wearing protective devices such as helmets, padding, and eyewear. Always buckle up when in cars.

- Have adequate first aid knowledge and skills. Even with the dramatic improvements to medical practice, the immediate attendance to injuries and illnesses often makes a difference in saving lives and preventing the further deterioration of the injury or illness.

- Obey the laws put in place to prevent injuries. This includes the laws on mandatory use of safety belts, the restrictions on the use of cell phones while driving, the requirement of the manufacturers to build airbags in cars, etc.

- Having a prepared action plan in cases of emergencies will help you act calmly in a stressful situation and take the proper steps instead of panicking.

Car Safety

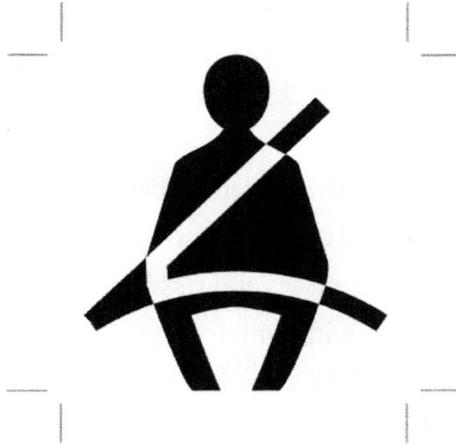

The emergency departments report that there are about 5 million car crash visits every year. Car related injuries and deaths cause a significant economic burden.

There are several vehicle safety practices, and they include:

- Do not drink and drive. Anyone planning on drinking alcohol should plan ahead and prepare an alternate means of transportation or take a taxi or public transportation. If in a group, assign a designated driver, someone, who agrees not to consume alcohol during the occasion.

- Avoid distractions and keep your eyes on the road. Anything that takes your eyes off the road, your mind off driving, or your hands off the wheel is dangerous and should be avoided. Making use of electronic devices such as text messaging or calling while driving could be disastrous. The use of electronic devices while behind the wheels have led to thousands of collisions and highway fatalities. Other distractions like eating, drinking, talking to passengers, operating the radios, CDs, or MP3 players can also lead to accidents.

- While in the car, always remember to use the seat belt. Even though most of the cars on the road are equipped with airbags, those airbags present several risks to small children; the sheer amount of force with which they are deployed can severely injure small children, even killing infants. Children under the age of 13 should sit in the back seats away from the airbags.

- Children and infants must always sit in the back seats of cars in their child approved safety seat. The safety seat must fit the appropriate child in terms of age and weight. Also, ensure that the safety seats are properly installed in the car.

Fire Safety

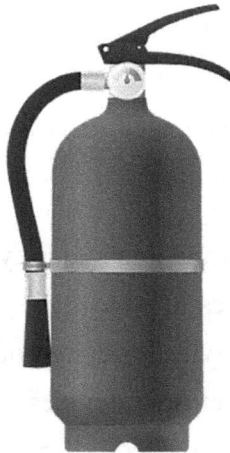

It is important to know what to do in cases of fire. Preventing fires and knowing what to do when fires do occur is important knowledge. About 3202 people died in 2006 from unintentional fires in the United States alone. About four out of ten deaths that occur from fires in homes without smoke alarms. To prevent fires, here are a few things that can be done.

- Let every floor of your home have its own smoke alarm. Check the batteries once a month and change them at least twice a year.

- Have fire extinguishers close by and matchsticks away from the reach of children.

- Keep flammable materials and space heaters away from the curtains.

- Fit guards around the fireplace, pipes, radiators, and wood-burning stoves.

However, being prepared in case of a fire incident reduces the risk of injuries or death. It is, therefore, important that there is a planned and precise escape plan for future use.

- Gather the family or roommates at a suitable time

- Prepare a sketch of the floor plans complete with the doors, windows, and hallways of every floor in the house.

- There should be two escape routes out of every room, especially the sleeping areas, because a lot of fire incidents occur at night.

- Prepare to make use of only the staircase

- Prepare a meeting spot for everyone outside the building

- Appoint an individual to make the necessary call to the fire department and which phone to use.

- Make sure everyone knows to leave the building first before calling for help.

The guidelines to follow to escape from a fire are:

- In the presence of smoke, crawl low to escape. This is because, during a fire, smoke rises, and the available breathable air is close to the floor.

- Children need to be taught how to open windows, climb down a ladder, and lower themselves onto the ground safely. There should be constant practice until the skill is perfected. Children must be out of the room first before the adults.

- Get out of the burning house quickly and do not return under any circumstance.

- If escape is impossible, stay in the room and stuff the door cracks and vents with wet towels, clothing, and rags. If there is a phone, call for help from the fire department, even if there are rescuers available outside, and let them know where you are.

- If you are in a hotel and you hear the fire alarm, touch your doorknob first. If the door is hot, do not go outside.

- The elevators should not be used. Make use of relatively smoke-free staircases instead.

- If the exit is not reachable, go back to your room and turn off the airing or ventilation system. The cracks in the door and vents should be stuffed with wet towels or clothing. Call the fire department immediately.

By following the safety procedures, you can prevent unintentional injuries that affect thousands of people every year and lead to a great deal of loss. Injuries do not just happen, and some steps can be taken to prevent them. Acquiring the knowledge on what to do in cases of incidents and accidents also helps in saving lives and preventing the deterioration of injuries.

Conclusion

First aid knowledge and skills are important. They are skills and knowledge that everyone should possess. Accidents happen daily; riots can break out even in the middle of a peaceful protest, a slip off the stairs, and a minute distraction while handling flammable substances can lead to emergencies requiring medical aid. The EMS personnel do not always arrive at once due to various circumstances beyond their control. With the first aid knowledge, you will be fully equipped to help save the lives of victims of accidents and injuries wherever you find yourself. With the full understanding of what is wrong with the victim, you are well equipped to take the appropriate steps towards saving the life of the victim and preventing the further deterioration of the injuries rather than just winging it.

Save a life. Learn first aid today. Thank you for reading.

FIRST AID
HANDBOOK

How to Heal from Domestic Accidents

BRANDA NURT

Introduction

Accidents are a common occurrence in our lives. They can occur in a variety of settings, from roads to the office, just to mention a few. One of the places where accidents easily occur is our homes. They can be a major cause of the discomfort, injury, or even deaths depending on how serious the accident was. They can also happen to people of all ages, but children and the elderly are the most prone to domestic accidents.

Since they are very common, it's worth knowing as much as possible about domestic accidents so that you can better handle them when they occur. Domestic accidents range from minor ones that only require some first aid treatment to major ones that would need the intervention of a medical practitioner.

No domestic accident is the same. There are several types of them all with different causes and symptoms to look out for. The methods of first aid used for the different types of accidents also differ, and so do the actual treatment processes. Some will take longer to heal, while some could take just a day if not a few hours. Some domestic accidents can affect not only our physical well-being but also our mental health if they are not treated properly or promptly.

It's also important to note that at the end of the day, even though they are very common and you can heal from most domestic accidents, it's better to be safe and avoid them altogether. They may be sudden, but there are certain things you could do to reduce the chances of these accidents happening in your home.

In this book, we discuss domestic accidents at length. In it, we talk about the common types of domestic accidents, how to prevent them, first aid for domestic accidents, further treatments, and how to heal from them.

Chapter 1

First Aid for Domestic Accidents

What is First Aid?

First Aid refers to the immediate response or assistance that you give to a person who just suffered an injury. First aid is usually administered to a victim to preserve their life and to stop their condition from getting worse. It also promotes faster recovery from injury or illness. It can be said that first aid is the first kind of intervention given before the victim gets professional help. In some cases, first aid may actually be the only intervention needed for the victim to feel better.

What is the Purpose of First Aid When a Domestic Accident Happens?

It is almost impossible to predict when accidents will take place. However, when one occurs, you must be ready to help, and first aid is the best way to go about it before you seek any professional help. The aims of first aid include:

Preserving Life

Remember that a first aider is not a medical professional. However, first aid ensures that a victim of a domestic accident gets basic care since first aid can treat minor injuries that do not need emergency attention or routine check-ups. That said, should the situation be more difficult to the extent that it threatens the patient's life, the focus of first aid is to preserve life long enough until the victim has access to professional care.

Preventing Escalation of the Situation

First aid is provided to prolong the time that the patient has before the ambulance arrives. For example, if there is profuse bleeding, the attention of the first aider is not going to be to stitch the wound, but rather to stop the bleeding so that the chances of further complications are reduced.

Relieving Pain

If you're a first aider and are uncertain about medications, it's better to ask a professional or avoid administering medication altogether.

Self-Protection

When administering first aid, you must protect yourself. Be sure the area and surroundings are safe. Don't try to be the "hero" and end up being a victim too.

Promoting Recovery

If you're administering first aid, your actions should be aimed towards helping the victim of the domestic accident get better faster. It means using your first aid kit and all its supplies to help the person.

What is Basic First Aid?

Basic first is made easy by the formula DRABC. Here is what that stands for:

D- Danger

Always look around to see if there's anything that could harm you or anyone else in the area whenever a domestic accident has happened. Then check if there's any danger to the injured person. The most important thing is that you avoid putting yourself in any kind of danger in the process of trying to assist someone.

R-Response

Check carefully whether the victim of the domestic accident is responsive or conscious. Does the person react when you call out to them or when you firmly touch or squeeze their hands or shoulder?

A-Airway

Check on the victim's airway. Is it clear? It's important to ensure that the person is actually breathing. In case the person does respond even if their airway has no barrier, find out ways in which you can assist them with their injury. If they do not respond and are unconscious, you must check their airway by doing the head-tilt and chin-lift maneuver, and opening their mouth looking inside.

To perform the head-tilt and chin-lift maneuver you must place one hand over the forehead and the other hand under the chin. Then carefully lift the chin and tilt the head back at the same time; be careful not to do sudden movements to avoid damage to the cervical spine. Once the neck's in an optimal position, you can search their mouth.

If you find that the inside of their mouth is clear, slowly continue by tilting their head back and check that they're actually breathing. If their mouth isn't clear, you could place them gently on the side and then sweep your finger through the victim's mouth so that you're able to clear all the unwanted contents in it. After that, you can perform the head-tilt chin-lift maneuver once again and recheck for breathing.

B-Breathing

Check keenly whether the person is breathing by observing their chest movement. Put your ear next to their mouth and then to their nose to listen. You should also place your hand on their chest, targeting the lower part to feel whether they are breathing. If you find that they are breathing even if they are unconscious, turn them to their side and be careful with their body position.

Make sure the victim's head, neck, and spine are aligned and make sure you keep track of their breathing at all times. If the person's breathing, you must measure the respiratory rate. This is done by counting the number of breaths in 20 seconds and multiplying it by three, and it's very valuable information for the medical team.

If the person isn't breathing, there's a chance that the heart's not beating either. If the person's heart isn't beating, you must provide Cardiopulmonary Resuscitation. If, however, the heart is beating, you must provide Breathing Cardiopulmonary Resuscitation to bypass the function of the lungs and provide oxygen to the person.

This is done with the person's back flat on the floor, you perform the head-tilt and chin-lift maneuver, breathe in some air, close the nose with your fingers, cover the mouth with your mouth and release air into the person's oral cavity. Blowing air into the person's mouth with this technique is called a rescue breath, and each rescue breath must last around one second. You should provide one rescue breath every five to six seconds until the person is breathing again, or until a health-care professional is around to take over the situation.

C- Circulation

Here, you must check the patient's circulatory status. This begins by taking the patient's pulse. The radial pulse and the carotid pulse are the easiest ones to locate and measure. The radial pulse is located in the wrist, below the thumb, and the carotid pulse is located in the neck, at either side of Adam's Apple. Gently place your index, middle, and ring fingers over either of these areas and feel the pulsations of the blood flowing. If you're able to feel the pulse, count how many pulsations happen in fifteen seconds and multiply that by four to get the pulse rate, also very important for the medical team.

If you don't feel the pulse, place your head over the person's chest to hear the heart beating. If you don't notice any heartbeats, then it's time to apply cardiopulmonary resuscitation.

First, make sure that they are lying on their back over a hard surface. They should be flat. Put one of the heels of either hand at the center part of the victim's chest, then place your second hand on top and press it down very firmly but smoothly about 30 times. The hands must descend at least 2 inches, but no more than 2.4 inches. After you're done with the 30 chest compressions, you must provide two rescue breaths, just as described in the Breathing Cardiopulmonary Resuscitation. This is called a cycle of CPR, composed of 30 chest compressions plus two rescue breaths. You should provide at least five cycles of CPR every 2 minutes until the heart starts beating again, or up to the time you finally get help from a trained professional.

Defibrillator

We can add a defibrillator into the process. This machine is meant to deliver an electric shock that will restore a normal heartbeat. They are easy to operate since all you need to do is follow the steps and the pictures on the package and the voice instructions. Once the victim responds, you should turn them to face the side and keep their head tilted so that ysou maintain a clear airway.

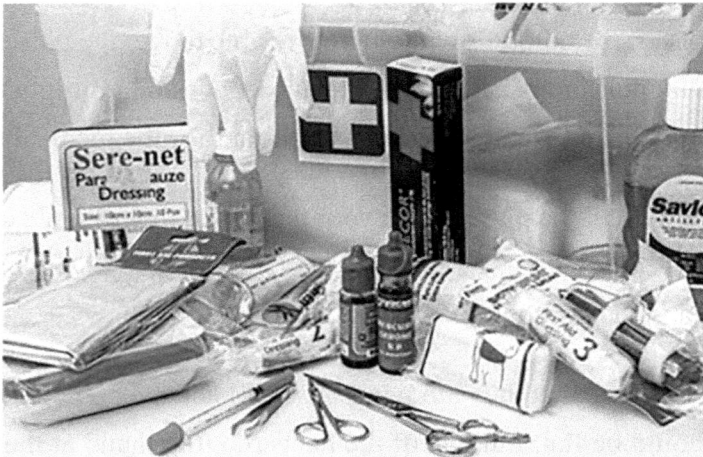

The Contents of a First Aid Kit

For you to administer first aid when there's a domestic accident, it's important to have a first aid kit. Some of the contents of a first aid kit include:

- Various bandages and gauze

- Adhesive tape

- Sterile gauze

- Eye pads

- Wet wipes

- Clasps and safety pins

- Antibiotic ointment

- Saline solution

- Scissors and tweezers

- A first aid guide

- CPR masks

- Disposable gloves

- A thermometer(digital ones are preferred)

- Skin rash cream

- Sprays to relieve insect bites

- Painkillers

- Antiseptic cream

- Distilled water to clean wounds

- Antihistamine creams or tablets

Importance of Learning First Aid

It is common for domestic accidents to happen, which is why first aid knowledge is very important. Here are some of the benefits of learning first aid.

It Helps Save Lives

There are different types of domestic accidents, as has already been mentioned, and some of them can be fatal if not managed immediately. Giving first aid can help reduce recovery time and goes a long way in determining whether the accident victim will have a temporary or even permanent disability. This is why it's so important to learn how to carry out first aid. You will, through first aid lessons, learn how to stay calm whenever there's a domestic accident and will be able also to learn simple acronyms that will help you remember the steps that you are required to take to help save the victim's life. First aid training is, therefore, important in helping you become more confident and comfortable in taking control of the situation when an accident occurs.

It Helps You Increase a Victim's Comfort

Not all domestic accidents will require that the patient be taken to a hospital. Through first aid training, you will know how to act by employing some simple techniques like using ice packs or tying bandages properly. You will also be prepared to make the patient emotionally comfortable.

First Aid Training Helps You Prevent the Situation from Worsening

Sometimes even domestic accidents could become worse if the victim doesn't receive basic first aid. Getting first aid training, therefore, means you will be able to keep a patient stable until the emergency medical help arrives at the scene of the domestic accident. First aid training will help you learn how to use basic items in your home as tools in case a first aid kit is not within reach, so you'll be able to deal with different accident situations. Through the training, you will also learn how best to collect information on how the accident happened so that you can effectively pass it to the professional medical practitioners.

First Aid Training Encourages Healthy Living and Safety within the House

When you decide to get first aid training, the first lesson you will learn is how to take care of yourself and how to ensure the safety of all those around you. Keeping yourself safe means you'll be better positioned to help other people.

It Gives You a Sense of Security

Learning about first aid makes you feel more secure as you're aware that in case of a domestic accident, you can even save your own life aside from the lives of those who are around you. It also makes those people who are close to you feel more secure, and it reassures them.

Origins of First Aid

It is said that St. John Ambulance was the first organization to incorporate the use of first aid in the year 1879 in the United Kingdom. Queen Victoria's daughter Princess Christian then translated five ambulance lectures that were delivered in German to English. Prof. Esmarch had given the lectures in 1882. These lectures were published with the title First Aid to the Injured. It was published by Smith Elder, who had help from a group of partners. In 1882, St. Andrew started the First Aid organization to help care for those who had been injured during the war and to give them any other form of care that they required. Sir George Beatson then wrote down the regulation of the organization. It was then issued in 1891.

In 1908, both the St. Andrew and St. John's organizations agreed to merge and carry out all their activities as one. Esmarch, between 1823 and 1908, created the foundation for first aid institutions that are more civil. He then became a physician in the year 1948 and later studied surgery.

Another version of the story says that first aid generally has a very complicated history. There isn't too much information on the pre-historic man, but they were certainly confronted with various situations that needed first aid. They probably came up with different ways to stop things like bleeding, ways to stabilize bones when they broke accidentally, and different ways to determine whether plants were poisonous or not.

Over time, different people became more knowledgeable and skillful in handling medical situations that they were faced with. They could have been witchdoctors or first shamans. This might have been the first stage of the distinction between the type of healthcare that could be provided by amateurs or laymen and healthcare that could be provided by professionals. It became clearer and clearer what they all could offer as medical training became more formal.

We also cannot mention first aid history without talking about the days of war whereby when people were in battles or wars and got injured, they would usually die whenever there was a lack of medical attention. In 1099 the religious knights got training on medical care. This training was organized by the order of St. John. It was training specifically on the treatment of injuries obtained from the battlefield.

In the mid-19th century, the First International Geneva Convention took place and led to the creation of the Red Cross organization to help the soldiers who were wounded from wars. Through this, soldiers received training on how to treat their colleagues before medics arrived to give further treatment.

After a decade, one of the army surgeons proposed that civilians should be trained in first aid, which he at the time called pre-medical treatment. The term first aid was first used back in 1878 as a combination of the phrases "first treatment" and "National Aid." Over time, the practical skills involved in first aid have evolved, and somehow, first aid is separated from emergency medicine. Today, even the ambulances that are called at the scene of accidents have personnel who are well trained on first aid and also have advanced training making them paramedics.

The First - First Aid Kit

In America, the First Aid Kit was inspired by a fateful conversation. It was called the Johnson and Johnson First Aid kit and was released for use in 1888. Robert Wood Johnson was on a train on the way to Colorado for a nice vacation when he started a conversation with the Rio Grande and Denver railway chief surgeon. The doctor started to explain the dangers of railroad construction. He went ahead to talk about the fact that there was a clear lack of medical supplies to give treatment to the industrial injuries that are often unique compared to many other types of injuries.

It was through this conversation on health that Johnson saw a great business opportunity. He already had a small business, and the idea he had in him at the time was also a way to advance his knowledge in healthcare. He, therefore, created the very first commercial first aid kit.

During the 19th century, those who worked in railway construction had to be taken to isolated areas on the Western side of America, which was so far away from hospitals and any other form of traditional healthcare. In 1869, the very first transcontinental railroad was constructed and completed in the same year. In the following years, expansion continued, and between the years 1880 and 1890, over 70000 miles of tracks were newly laid.

This expansion project in the rural areas that were so rugged meant that the workers were constantly prone to dangerous conditions, and accidents were very common. Whenever disaster struck, accidents would end up fatal. During these times, the death rate of then workers stood at 12,000 every year. Incorporating cutting edge machinery in the construction exposed them to new kinds of injuries, yet there was no form of medical care to assist in such situations.

Working on the steam locomotives also posed a great threat to people to the extent that trains began carrying surgeons on board. They also started to carry medical vehicles to offer medical assistance to these workers. In the 1800s, along the stretch between the states of Louisiana, Missouri and Texas, there wasn't a single hospital. This was a 1300-mile stretch, which would explain why so many people died in the process.

Railroad companies decided to employ their own medical practitioners to handle such situations. The practitioners had to learn everything about surgery while already on the job and had to improvise care for trauma along the way. They found different ways to deal with the new kinds of injuries the workers got, especially those that involved crushed limbs. They came up with new technologies in healthcare and sterile surgery.

Despite this, it was hard to put theory into practice, and it was even harder to keep germs away from wounds. The railway medical practitioners, therefore, championed the building of hospitals, but the death rate remained extremely high. It's then that it was discovered that what was lacking the entire time were educated people to serve as first responders and also antiseptics to help give the first aid to injured workers.

The workers would naturally help their fellow workers whenever they would get injured but were untrained and had very little knowledge of basic hygiene or how to care for the wounds. Due to this, their attempts brought more harm to the victims than good. It is then that Robert Wood Johnson came up with a solution.

Wood invented the Johnson and Johnson's surgical products that were sterile and were placed in boxes that could stay with the railway workers in case of any injuries. He wrote to the railway medical practitioners and asked them what they needed to have in those kits. He then had them translated into products by his company's scientific director known as Fred Kilmer, a very experienced pharmacist. Thanks to his meticulous research, the first-ever First Aid Kit was developed in 1888. The company's kits were well packed in either metal or wooden boxes and included surgical products like adhesive plasters, gauzes, dressing bandages, plasters, and sutures.

These kits would bridge the gap between the injuries and the treatment required. Kilmer understood the workers also needed some training on how to treat the injuries with the help of the kits. As such, in 1901, the Johnson & Johnson Company created and published a book to help with this. It was called the Hand Book of First Aid. It was very comprehensive and was commercially available, something which allowed it to reach many more people aside from just railway workers. It taught them basic hygiene and also emergency care. It gave people directions on how to use Johnson and Johnson products. This actually sparked a movement, and with time, many more guides similar to Kilmer's were developed. First Aid Kits then increased in popularity with different people or companies coming up with their own.

Within a short time, just a decade, it became part of the law in 1910 that any workplace in America with over three employees needed to have a First Aid Kit. Throughout the rest of the century, the kits were improved to meet the new needs in terms of medical care. Companies started customizing them for schools, the workplace and homes depending on the kinds of injuries people were susceptible to while there. Today, the Johnson& Johnson kits remain the standard when it comes to offering emergency care.

Chapter 2

Types of Domestic Accidents
and Prevention

What is a Domestic Accident?

A domestic accident is an accident that takes place within your home and its immediate surroundings. Domestic accidents happen everywhere in the world and are a major source of concern. In some countries, in fact, these accidents that happen at home kill more people compared to other types of accidents regardless of all the safety regulations that many people follow. The problem is even worse in developing countries where some people live under deplorable conditions.

Any kind of accident is usually a source of distress to the victim and the people around them. Accidents can have minor consequences or major ones in some situations whereby the entire community could feel the effects. Some can lead to disability, either temporary or permanent.

It goes without saying that children are the most susceptible when it comes to home accidents since they often do not notice that certain things pose a threat to them. In some cases, they are unable to read, which results in accidents such as poisoning since they confuse certain poisonous substances for consumables.

Types of Domestic Accidents

There are many types of domestic accidents. They include:

Falling Objects

This is a common type of domestic accident, especially in homes that have children who have just started to move around without assistance. Children can pull things over onto them, such as a dresser, tv, or even a stove. They also tend to grab and pull at things over their head, which can lead to disaster, like pulling a table cloth, with dishes and hot food tumbling down.

Prevention

You can prevent accidents from falling objects by ensuring there are no loose wires, electrical leads, dish towels, tablecloth edges, and the likes nearby. Make sure they are completely away from your children's reach. Remember, however, that just because children are the most susceptible to accidents doesn't mean grown-ups aren't also.

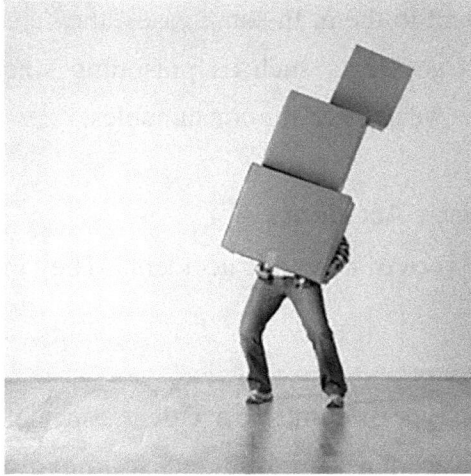

Accidents from Falls

Another common type of domestic accident is trips or falls. These affect people of all ages, whether children or adults. Some of the common causes of falling accidents include:

- Uneven floors or surfaces

- Floors that have been recently waxed or mopped

- Floorboards that have been loosely placed, rugs, and mats

- Poor lighting

- Open desks or drawers

- Cords running across walkways

- The glare from bright lights

- Lack of handrails on staircases

- Going up and down staircases in a rush

- Using a ladder that's not being held by someone or one that's not secured

- Using furniture instead of a ladder for climbing

Sprains

Sprains occur when the ligaments which connect your joints are stretched, twisted, or even torn. They mostly occur around your knees, wrists, or ankles. Some of the causes of sprains in the home include:

- Walking or running on surfaces that are uneven in your home

- Suddenly twisting your joints or pivoting

- Falls whereby you land on your hand or wrist

- Throwing something forcefully

- Injuries from indoor exercising or sports at home

Burns

Unfortunately, there are countless items in the home area that could cause nasty burns. Such items include cooking pans, ovens, kettles, and other cooking ranges. Some people also have other items such as matches, hair strengtheners, lawnmowers, and radiators that are known to cause burns. And don't forget sunburns, which are very common, but preventable.

Types of Burns

Burns are categorized according to the extent of the injury.

- First-Degree Burns: These are burns that involve the top or outermost layer of the skin. This layer of your skin is called the epidermis. This type of burn has a red appearance and is tender and painful. The burns could also lead to swelling. First degree burns are usually not categorized by blisters and heal quickly. This kind of burn often occurs from over-exposure to the sun's harmful UV rays or when you come into contact with a hot object.

- Second-Degree Burns: Second-degree burns are those that affect the second layer of the skin. This layer is called the dermis. These kinds of burns have a pink appearance and are usually soft and moist. They are very painful and are characterized by blisters. The blisters contain fluid that might end up oozing from the skin. Depending on the extent of damage, they may take between two to six weeks to heal. They may leave a scar.

- Third-Degree Burns: Third-degree burns involve damage to three layers of the skin. They are the epidermis, the dermis, and also the hypodermis. With this type of burn, your skin's full layer is damaged. Fat, nerves, muscles, and even bones could end up being affected. This kind of skin damage causes the skin to develop a white filmy appearance. With these burns, the victim will experience tremendous pain because of the damage caused to the nerve endings. Third-degree burns are often caused by fires, corrosive chemicals, or electricity.

If you believe the burns are third degree burns, seek medical attention immediately or call 911 immediately!

Prevention of Burns

These are the general measures you'll have to follow personally and at home to prevent burns.

- Install smoke alarms and make sure that they're working properly.

- Make sure that you have at least one fire extinguisher and learn how to use it properly.

- Make evacuation plans in case of a fire. Find the emergency exits, as well as any other auxiliary last-resource exits (such as windows), and memorize them.

- Make sure to check the electrical wiring of your home with a professional electrician at least once every ten years.

- If you have a fireplace, have it inspected and cleaned at least once a year with a professional.

- Make sure to wear sunscreen, especially days and places such as the beach.

- Hot seat-belts and straps have the capacity to provoke second-degree burns on infants and small children, so make sure that you check whether these are hot or not before getting a child inside a car. If these are too hot, use a towel to keep the infant's skin from burning.

- Make sure that you wear gloves when you handle hazardous chemicals to prevent chemical burns.

- Keep inflammable objects such as matches and lighters locked up, away from children.

- Prevent electrical burns in children by covering all electrical outlets.

- Don't let children close to any source of fire or heat such as kitchen stoves.

- Space heaters must be at least three feet away from any inflammable objects such as curtains and rugs. Make sure that children stay away from them.

- Don't let candles unattended, and if you smoke, make sure to turn off the cigar before disposing of it.

- Make sure not to store inflammable materials unless it's necessary. Dry weeds and leaves have no reason to be kept at home, and they represent a risk of fire.

- Make sure that the baby milk is at the right temperature, and don't heat baby bottles in microwave ovens for that reason, because they tend to heat things unevenly.

- Make sure to put out the small fires of the stoves by sliding a lid over the fire.

- Things such as hot irons must be unplugged after use, and they must be kept away from children.

- Don't cook wearing something with long-loose sleeves.

- Make sure that the handles of the pans and pots away from you to avoid flipping them over by mistake.

Inhalation Burns

These types of burns can make your airway swell and make it harder for you to breathe. With inhalation burns, you must seek emergency medical care immediately. The symptoms of these burns can progress quickly and a person's ability to breathe can be severely compromised.

Choking

Choking happens when an object, piece of food, or liquid causes blockage in the throat. Many times children will choke after placing a foreign object into their mouth. Adults can also choke while eating or drinking, especially if they're doing it rapidly.

It's common for people to choke because it's often short-lived and does not pose any kind of danger. However, sometimes choking is life-threatening when the object or gets stuck in the throat and cuts off the air supply.

Poisoning

Poisoning accidents at home are very dangerous and should be managed immediately. Some of the common causes of poisoning include:

- Medication, especially painkillers. Other, unexpected medications such as steroid creams and cough medicine can contribute to an overdose. Children are especially at risk as pills can look like candy. However, these medications do not have to be in pill form. They can also come in adhesive patches that could stick on a child's skin, or a child might end up sucking on them.

- Some cleaning products including disinfectant, bleach, caustic soda, among others. Poisoning from these especially, among children can lead to damage to the airway or gastrointestinal tract.

- Some of the products used for DIY projects such as glue, wallpaper paste, and paint.

- Different cosmetics such as shampoos, nail varnish remover, and baby oil.

- Some of the products you use in the garden such as rat poison and weed killer.

- Some types of plants could also cause poisoning when eaten. In some cases, the effects are mild, but in some cases, it can be very serious. If you require emergency treatment, take a few leaves from the plant to the emergency room with you.

- Food that has mold, not cleaned properly, or undercooked meat.

- Carbon monoxide, which is an odorless and colorless gas that can be deadly. It is produced from burning fuels like wood, gas, and petrol. It may also be produced by appliances that are not functioning properly. Those appliances include gas ranges, space heaters, portable generators, stoves, and wood-burning fireplaces. When carbon monoxide is in low concentration, it causes flu-like symptoms like fatigue, headache, and nausea. When it's in high concentration, it can lead to difficulty in breathing, loss of consciousness, coma, and even worse, death.

- Alcohol, nicotine, and other illicit substances could also cause poisoning. If you have children in your house, they can get alcohol intoxication if they accidentally end up drinking alcoholic beverages like wine, beer, and alcohol. Perfumes, mouthwashes, and hand sanitizers also contain alcohol that can cause poisoning, seizures and could even lead to coma when ingested by children. The type of liquid nicotine solution that's used in e-cigarettes can also poison a child when they accidentally ingest it or when it comes into contact with their skin. Cigarettes, chewing tobacco, and nicotine gum can also be poisonous. Nicotine patches can be poisonous to children and can cause nausea, seizures, or vomiting. Illicit substances are also known to cause poisoning and many other serious health effects that include a change in alertness, responsiveness, and a change in breathing. These substances include methamphetamine, cocaine, synthetic cannabinoids, etc.

- Hydrocarbons such as kerosene, gasoline, lighter fluid, lamp oil paint thinners, and motor oil.

- Batteries or items that operate on batteries such as remote controls, calculators, toys, and watches. Younger children can accidentally swallow these batteries, especially the flat button-shaped ones. Batteries contain chemicals that are alkaline in nature and can leak or may generate an electric current that could end up burning them or creating holes in the esophagus.

Those are just a few causes of poisoning at home, but you can prevent poisoning accidents in the following ways.

Poison Prevention

- Ensuring that your fuel-burning appliances, for example, the electric fires and heaters around your house are well maintained and serviced on a regular basis.

- Keep the rooms that hold your appliances well ventilated and ensure you have a carbon monoxide detectors in your home.

- Ensure your air vents, chimneys, and flues are not blocked. If you like indoor fires, make sure you only have them in rooms that are well ventilated.

- Take a closer look at your home garden and examine the plants. Check whether the leaves, flowers, berries or the fruits of certain plants are poisonous and take the necessary precautions.

- Items like barbecue fuel, methylated spirits, weed killers and fertilizers should be kept in the garage or locked garden shed.

- If you need to burn rubbish, do not burn plastics, treated wood, old chemical tins or certain plants that are known to emit poisonous gases. Check your local laws. Some areas require a burn permit.

- Keep medication out of reach and locked away. Store cleaning products and chemicals in cabinets that are lockable.

- Never store cleaning products, medicine or other chemicals that could be poisonous near food.

- Keep chemicals in the containers they came in and never put chemicals or medicines in a different container.

- Avoid mixing chemicals because it can result in the emission of poisonous fumes, which can be deadly. For instance, when bleach and ammonia are mixed together, it creates a toxic gas that can cause chemical burns to the lungs and eyes; it can be deadly.

- Stay away from areas that have been recently sprayed with fertilizers or pesticides.

Drowning

Drowning is defined as death through suffocation because of being submerged in water. If someone is rescued from drowning, but that person inhaled water and was close to dying, then the person's health is still in danger. This is called near-drowning, which can be defined as surviving after suffocation provoked by being submerged in water. Near-drowning experiences can end up being fatal or carry further complications in the future if medical attention is not immediately provided to the victim.

Common Causes of Drowning

- Inability to swim.

- Panicking and fatigue are common causes of drowning.

- Unattended children. When children are swimming, they should always be supervised by responsible adults, even when the child knows how to swim. Just one moment of distraction and a child can slip under the water and drown.

- Unattended baths. Drowning does not only occur in swimming pools but can also happen in the bathroom. When your child is in the bath, you should stay with them in the bathroom until they are done. Just a couple minutes away can have tragic results. Stay with them until the water is drained.

- While many drowning accidents happen in the summertime, some can happen during the winter, such as when one falls through the ice.

- Swimming while intoxicated.

- Heart attacks, concussions, and seizures in the water can also cause drowning.

- Suicide attempts such as jumping from a bridge.

- Diving injuries.

- Flash floods. Don't drive through high standing water. Remember the saying – "Don't drown. Turn around."

- Remember to keep toilet bowls covered. A lot of people think that drowning only occurs in large bodies of water, but it can actually in small amounts of water.

Heart Attacks (Myocardial Infarction)

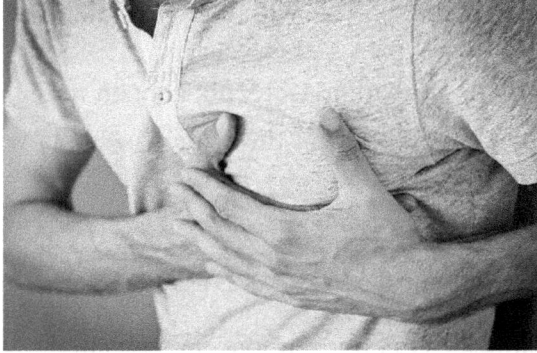

A heart attack, also known as Myocardial Infarction, is the death of part of the muscular tissue of the heart due to a lack of blood flow. This usually happens when one of the arteries nurturing the heart, the coronary arteries, is blocked, or the body becomes unable to carry oxygen. Atherosclerosis is the most common cause for Myocardial Infarction; in this disease, fatty deposits are formed in the inner walls of the arteries. Arteries affected can be easily clogged and obstructed by an embolus (an unattached mass flowing through the blood vessels, most likely a piece of a blood clot). A fatty deposit can also be broken, forming a blood clot that will ultimately obstruct the coronary artery, causing the heart attack.

If you believe a heart attack is occurring call 911!

Prevention of a Heart Attack

Since they're such a predominant and lethal syndrome, almost all healthy habits are directed towards preventing heart attacks. So, it's fair to say that living a healthy life will prevent heart attacks; the common recommendations include:

352

- Not smoking.

- Drinking less.

- No illicit drugs.

- Regular exercise (especially cardiovascular exercise).

- Low-sodium, low-sugar, and low-cholesterol diet.

- Having a healthy body weight.

- Stress management.

- Treatment of any underlying diseases (especially hypertension, Diabetes Mellitus, and hypercoagulable disorders).

This last recommendation is extremely important in the prevention of heart attacks, and will also help you think about them whenever you see symptoms that are similar to those of a heart attack—obesity, smoking, alcoholism, hypertension, diabetes mellitus, hypercoagulable disorders - these are all factors associated with heart attacks. Their presence facilitates the diagnosis and should always be treated and reduced as much as possible to prevent Myocardial Infarctions from happening.

Stroke

A stroke is a similar syndrome to a heart attack, but instead of the heart muscle, it happens in the brain tissue. A stroke is an interruption of the blood flow to a part of the brain, either because of an obstruction or a rupture of an artery (or group of arteries). Strokes are very dangerous because they can easily leave life-long consequences, or even be lethal.

If you believe a stroke is occurring call 911!

Stroke Prevention

Since a stroke is just a heart attack that happens in a different place, preventing a stroke is very similar to preventing a Myocardial Infarction.

- Healthy low-sugar, low-sodium, and low-cholesterol diet.

- Regular exercise.

- Healthy weight.

- Avoid smoking and illegal drugs.

- Reduce alcohol consumption.

- Treat any associated underlying diseases such as Diabetes Mellitus, obesity, and hypercoagulable disorders.

Kidney Stones (Nephrolithiasis)

Nephrolithiasis, commonly known as kidney stones, is the obstruction of the renal ducts, which are the channels through which urine travels from the kidneys to the bladder. Once the renal ducts are obstructed, the urine starts to accumulate in the kidney, causing infections and other complications.

Identifying Kidney Stones

Unless viewed by a physician during a routine check, kidney stones will stay inside the kidney without causing symptoms until they move to the renal ducts and obstruct them. Then, the person starts to experience extreme discomfort that manifests mainly with pain. Nephrotic pain is sharp and it comes in waves of varying intensity, but it's usually very intense. It's mainly located in the lower back, but it can also go to the lower abdomen and groin. Other symptoms associated with kidney stones are:

- Vomiting and nausea.

- Blood in the urine.

- A persistent need to urinate.

- Dark urine, foul-smelling urine, and/or fever if an infection has developed.

Preventing Kidney Stones

It's said that a kidney that creates kidney stones will always create them; this is because there's an important genetic factor associated with Nephrolithiasis. However, there are many aspects of life we can change to reduce the risk of developing a kidney stone.

- Stay hydrated.

- Have a low-fat, low-animal protein, and especially a low-sodium diet.

- Healthy body weight.

Gallbladder Attack (Biliary Obstruction)

The gallbladder is a hollow organ responsible for storing and liberating bile into the intestine. It's located inside the liver and it delivers the bile through channels called bile ducts. The liver shares this task with the gallbladder, producing bile on its own and releasing it into the intestine through its own bile duct (that merges with the gallbladder's bile duct before reaching the intestine). Whenever the bile ducts are obstructed, usually by gallstones, you have developed a biliary obstruction. Biliary obstruction is a painful syndrome that can get complicated with infections (especially when it's caused by one). It's clinically hard to differentiate a biliary obstruction from other diseases such as appendicitis, and especially pancreatitis, so you should always go to a physician anytime you see these symptoms (admittedly, the pain will usually urge you to seek medical assistance).

Identifying a Biliary Obstruction

Symptoms can be acute if the obstruction is sudden or chronic and progressive if the obstruction is a slow process taking place. The most salient symptom is abdominal pain. This severe pain will typically be located in the upper right side of the abdomen under the rib cage. Another very important symptom that's very particular of biliary obstruction is yellowing of the eyes (icterus) and the skin (jaundice), dark-colored urine and light-colored stools. Other symptoms associated to biliary obstruction are:

- Generalized itching in the skin.

- Fever.

- Vomiting and nausea.

- Diminished appetite.

- Weight loss.

Preventing Biliary Obstruction

The most common gallstones that cause biliary obstruction are made of cholesterol, so a healthy weight and a good low-cholesterol high-fiber diet will reduce the risk of biliary obstruction. Also, extreme weight-loss diets of under 800 calories of daily intake should be avoided as they're also associated with biliary obstruction.

Asthma Attacks

Asthma is a chronic inflammatory lung disease that causes breathing problems. It's the most common chronic disease among children in America, and it can cause severe distress, as well as complications. Basically what happens in asthma is that the airways inside the lungs become inflamed, so they narrow down and get filled with mucus, making it harder for air to leave the lungs, forcing the person to gasp for breath as the body's oxygen levels drop. As the air struggles to leave the lungs, it shoots out the narrowed airways like a whistle, which causes the "wheezing" sound perceived in asthma during exhales. Asthma is both a chronic and episodic disease. Persons who have asthma will experience chronic symptoms, and they will get more severe in acute episodes called asthma attacks.

Identifying an Asthma Attack

A person suffering from an asthma attack will have trouble breathing; in particular inhalations will be short and desperate, while exhales will be longer (the air has trouble leaving the lungs, and then there's no space to fill with new air during inhales). The person will also exhibit the characteristic wheezing, a whistling sound during exhales that's sometimes so loud it can be heard without a stethoscope. Cough, tightness in the chest, anxiousness, fatigue, and pale or blue fingernails, face, or lips are also signs and symptoms of an asthma attack (the last ones, severe symptoms that should be taken more seriously).

Asthma Triggers

Asthma attacks don't appear at random, but instead, they have different triggers according to the type of asthma that affects the person:

- Allergic Asthma: Very common in children, this type of asthma is triggered by allergens such as pollen, mold, dust, pet dander, and anything that creates an allergic reaction in the person.

- Nonallergic Asthma: A little bit harder to control than allergic asthma, non-allergic asthma is triggered by extreme weather conditions and strong smells. So, triggers include cold weather, raindrops drenching, air pollution, burning wood, cigarette smoke, cleaning products, perfumes, and even stress or viral infections.

- Exercise-induced Bronchoconstriction: Previously known as exercise-induced asthma, this condition is triggered by any form of physical exercise.

- Occupational Asthma: Triggered by lung-irritators found in the workplace. These can be industrial chemicals, gas, fumes, dust, dyes, and rubber latex.

Preventing Asthma

Asthma is mostly a genetic disease, so it's difficult to prevent its development. However, a particular form of asthma, allergic asthma, can be prevented by keeping a good and healthy diet for babies and toddlers. Following the physician's recommendations for a healthy diet (such as avoiding meat, fish, and cereals at a young age) will keep allergens out of the diet, reducing the chance to develop allergies, and therefore, allergic asthma.

Once asthma has been developed, preventing an asthma attack is as simple as identifying the allergens and avoiding them. As a general rule, you should avoid smoke, cold weather, rain, and strong smells.

Suffocation and SIDS

If choking is asphyxia due to an object obstructing the windpipe, and drowning is asphyxia due to inhalation of liquid while under water, suffocation is asphyxia because there's a large object covering the person's face, or the environment of the person is left out without oxygen. It's uncommon to find yourself in an environment without oxygen accidentally, such conditions are present in underground, sealed, and out-of-orbit spaces. So, in either of these cases, following the regular safety measures should be enough to stay alive and healthy.

It's also uncommon to have your nose and mouth accidentally covered by an object that won't allow breathing. However, there's a particular group of people that's vulnerable to accidental suffocation; we're talking about babies under 1 year old, and the Sudden Infant Death Syndrome.

Sudden Infant Death Syndrome

This is a condition where babies under 1 year of age die unexpectedly. They're often found dead in their cribs, and the diagnosis is made once an investigator and an autopsy is conducted and no discernible cause of death is identified. Most of these cases are due suffocation since it's very difficult to find this in the investigation and autopsy.

Preventing Suffocation and SIDS

Most babies who die due suffocation do so in the night while they're sleeping.. There are many paths to take to avoid babies from accidentally suffocating in their sleep.

- Always put the baby to sleep on their backs: Babies that sleep on their stomachs are in danger of suffocating.

- Avoid sharing beds with babies: A baby sleeping with a larger person, such as a sibling, a parent, or any other family member is in danger of being accidentally covered and suffocated during sleep.

- Avoid stuffed animals, cribs, and pillows that are too soft: Softer surfaces are more likely to cover and seal the baby's face, causing suffocation.

Recommendations to avoid SIDS unrelated to suffocation are to avoid overheating the baby or the baby's room during the night, avoid smoking through pregnancy, and breastfeed the baby.

Head Injury

Head injuries can be defined as any form of trauma applied to the scalp, skull, or brain. Depending on the force of the trauma, head injuries can be really dangerous because they can compromise the brain, the most important and delicate organ of the human body.

Any form of trauma to the head should be studied by a physician, especially if there are neurological manifestations such as trouble to walk, intense headaches, and other signs and symptoms that will be covered in chapter eleven.

If you believe there is a serious head injury call 911!

Preventing Head Injuries

These recommendations are relevant for adults and infants.

- Drive safely: This means that you should respect traffic signals, wear your seat belts and never drive under the influence of alcohol.

- Use helmets: Helmets must be worn in any activities that require them such as going through a construction site and riding a bicycle.

- Create a safe environment at home: Install handrails in bathrooms and stairways, bathroom and shower floors should have non-slip mats, remove tripping hazards, and make sure that the lighting is enough. If there are small children at home, you should install corner and edge bumpers, safety locks at windows, safety gates at the stairways, and set a shock-absorbing floor in their playground.

Broken Bones

A fracture, commonly known as broken bones, is a condition in which there's a partial or complete break in the continuity of the bone. Accidental fractures are caused by severe traumatisms such as car accidents, falling from high places, and violent incidents. However, it's also possible to have a bone break due to a normal daily movement if there are underlying diseases that debilitated the bone.

Preventing Fractures

Other than the usual measurements for accident and violent events preventions and precautions, there are a couple of recommendations to make bones less prone to fractures.

- Eat a healthy diet: Especially with vegetables full of calcium.

- Exercise regularly: In this case, it's important to avoid violently raising the intensity of the exercise or else you risk developing stress fractures.

- Be aware of underlying diseases: Cancer, osteoporosis, and osteomyelitis are some of the conditions able to debilitate your bones.

REMEMBER: If you're in a life-threatening or emergency medical situation, seek medical assistance immediately.

Chapter 3

Cuts and Basic First Aid

Cuts are types of wounds where a sharp object separates the tissue. Accidents with sharp objects will often result in cuts, so it's important to know what to do with one of them.

Classification

Just like any other wounds, cuts can be classified according to their thickness in superficial, partial-thickness and full-thickness cuts.

Superficial

These cuts only reach the epidermis, which is the first layer of the skin. You'll recognize the epidermis as the thin leathery tissue that's over the skin. Superficial cuts don't need stitches.

Partial Thickness

These cuts involve the epidermis and dermis, the second layer of the skin. The dermis is a highly vascularized tissue, so it's going to be red with blood. This is how you'll recognize these cuts, as their content will be the red tissue of the skin. Partial-thickness cuts may or may not need stitches; it depends on many other factors that will be studied later.

Full Thickness

These cuts involve the epidermis, dermis, subcutaneous tissue, and everything below that. Subcutaneous tissue is the last layer of skin, and it's mainly composed of fat. All full-thickness cuts will need stitches, so if the content of the cut is fat, muscles, bones, or any other internal structure, you'll need to see a physician.

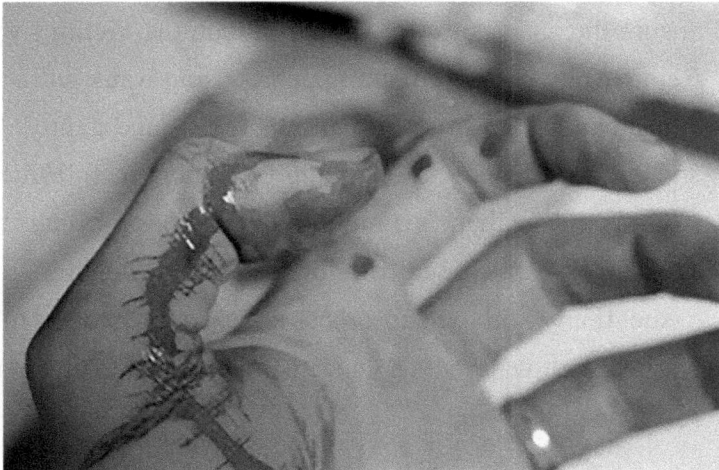

First Aid for Cuts

Most cuts can be treated at home, and whether it needs medical assistance or not, these are the first steps you should follow to treat a cut at home:

1. Wash your hands first so that you avoid any infections on the cut area

2. Ensure that you stop the bleeding completely. Usually, minor cuts will stop bleeding on their own, but if they do not, you can apply pressure gently on the cut area and use a clean gauze bandage or piece of cloth to elevate the victim's wound until the bleeding stops. If the bleeding doesn't stop after 15 minutes of pressure, or if the bleeding is too large, it'll need stitches.

3. Carefully clean the wound by rinsing it with clean water. Wash the area around the wound using some gentle soap but ensure the soap does not actually touch the victim's wound. Remove any dirt or remaining debris using water and a sterile gauze bandage to brush the dirt off the wound gently. Iodine and hydrogen peroxide shouldn't be used in full-thickness wounds unless there's a high risk of infection because these substances can cause irritation and delay healing in deep tissue. If any of these substances are used, the wound must be washed with water and a gauze bandage used to clean off the substance.

4. Apply an antibiotic ointment to the wound to keep the surface moist. You could notice some rashes appearing where the ointment has been applied. In such cases, you are advised to stop using the ointment. Petroleum jelly is restricted to superficial and partial thickness wounds.

5. Cover the wound properly using rolled gauze, a bandage, or use a gauze that has been properly held with paper tape.

Covering the victim's wound ensures it remains clean and protects it from infection.

6. Regularly change the dressing. Every time you change the dressing, take that chance to clean the wound once again. Doing it every day is best as it ensures the wound remains clean, and the person will also feel comfortable with the dressing. Nobody likes the feeling of a wet bandage, right?

7. Watch for any signs of infection on the wound or the skin near the wound. If there are signs of infection, a physician should be consulted to inspect the wound and apply antibiotics.

When to See a Doctor

A cut will need professional help to heal if it's bleeding profusely, it's infected (or in danger of infection), or if it needs stitches.

Stitches

As it has been described before, full-thickness wounds will always need stitches. Regarding partial thickness cuts, these are the rules you could follow.

- If there are cosmetic concerns regarding the cut, it will always need stitches. This includes all cuts to the face or neck and any other cuts that the person may wish to have treated without leaving a mark.

- Cuts with ragged edges will need stitches.

- Cuts that don't close by themselves will need stitches because they're an infection risk. This is especially true for cuts located in highly movable parts such as hands, fingers, and joints.

- The bleeding doesn't stop after applying pressure for 15 minutes.

- Wounds deeper than one-quarter of an inch that is also longer than three-quarters of an inch.

Signs of Infection

You should always see a doctor if a dirty object makes the wound. Examples of objects are rusty shards of metal, rusty metal wires, and anything that you may have a reason to think bacteria infects it. If a dirty object hasn't made the cut, there's still a chance that it may get infected, in which case you'll need to see a doctor. These are the signs that a cut may be infected:

- Pus coming out of the wound.

- The area could turn reddish, and this redness could spread. At first, it's quite normal to see redness. However, it should start to decrease, but if it does not within five days to a week, it could be a sign of infection.

- The pain could increase in the area of the wound

- You could feel sickly generally or even fatigued. You should generally feel better every day. However, if you do not, and instead feel fatigued or a lack of your usual energy, it could be a sign of infection.

- You could have fevers.

- Swollen glands

- Hot skin near your wound. Sometimes the area near the wound can feel warmer. Vasoactive chemicals have been released that increase the flow of blood to the area. The victim's immune system starts generating more heat by sending lymphocytes that facilitate the production of antibodies meant to destroy the infection-causing pathogens.

Chapter 4

Burns and Basic First Aid

B urns are common accidents, especially in the kitchen, so it's important to know how to deal with them.

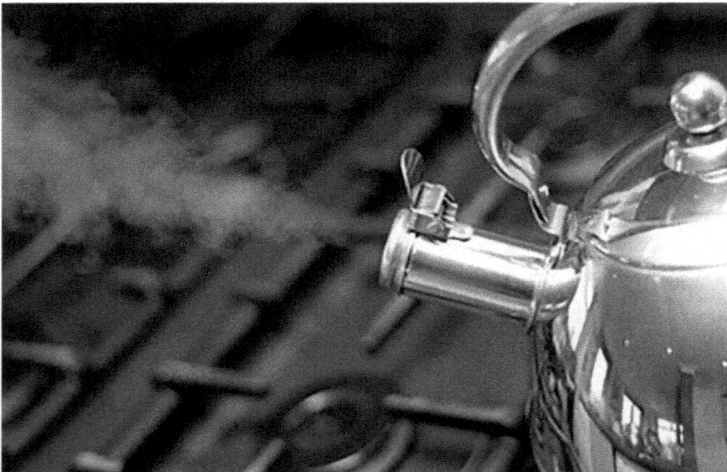

Symptoms from Burns

- Blisters

- Pain. You should note, however, that the amount of pain the victim will feel is not in any way related to how severe the burn is. This is because sometimes, the most severe burns have the least pain or no pain at all.

- Skin could start to peel.

- Your skin could also have a red appearance.

- Burn injury victims could experience shock so their skin could appear pale and clammy. Their lips and nails could turn bluish. They could also appear weak, and there may be a decrease in consciousness (the person becomes less alert).

- There may be swelling and inflammation in the burned area.

- The skin in the area could appear either white or charred.

- Their heart's rhythm could be disturbed in case the burn was caused by electricity.

Symptoms According to the Classification of Burns

Wounds are classified according to the extension of the damage they produced in the body. This allows us to identify the more severe burns, prioritize treatment, and treat them differently (not all burned wounds are treated the same). Depending on the affected skin layer (just like the rest of the wounds), burns are divided into first-degree (superficial), second-degree (partial thickness), and third-degree (full thickness) burns.

First-Degree Burns

These burns affect only the epidermis. They don't affect the dermis or anything below it. The usual example of a first-degree burn is the mild sunburn people with vulnerable skin get on the beach. The symptoms for these burns are red skin, pain, the wound is dry, and it has no blisters.

Second-Degree Burns

These burns reach the dermis layer. Second-degree burns are similar to first-degree burns, but they're much more painful and they develop blisters. These are also more dangerous than first-degree burns; if taken care of the wrong way, second-degree burns are prone to infections. The symptoms are pain, red skin, swelling, and blisters.

Third-Degree Burns

These burns completely destroy the epidermis, being able to reach everything below that skin layer, such as the subcutaneous tissue, tendons, muscles, and even bones. These wounds usually reach so far in the tissue that they destroy the nerves, so there's no sensitivity in the burned area; this means that these burns usually aren't painful. Since the burned area doesn't have an epidermis or dermis, the wound usually doesn't have the red color; instead; instead, the burned area will have a black, white, brown, or yellow color.

It's important to point out that most burned areas will exhibit several types of burns. This is because the different areas of the skin will interact differently with the burned area. A third-degree burn will usually be surrounded by second-degree burns, for example. You should follow the different first-aid recommendations for the types of wounds, prioritizing the most serious ones.

First Aid for Burns

If someone gets a burn accident, here's how to help them before emergency help arrives:

Major Burns

These are the steps you should follow for third-degree burns.

1. Protect the burn victim from further harm by getting them away from the cause of the burn. In case the cause of the burn is electrical, ensure that the power is off before you even move close to the victim so that you also don't put yourself in harm's way.

2. Ensure the victim is still breathing. If they are not, start rescue breathing and call 911. If the person's heart isn't beating, start CPR.

3. Take off any jewelry and restrictive items such as belts from the victim, especially if it's around the neck area or the burned area.

4. Cover the burnt area using a cool bandage that's moist or grabs a clean piece of cloth and covers the area with it.

5. Avoid immersing severe burns in water as this could lead to a loss in body heat, a condition known as hypothermia.

6. Keep the burnt area elevated. If possible, above the level of the victim's heart.

7. Check for any signs of shock. Signs and symptoms for this usually include fainting, slow breathing or a pale complexion.

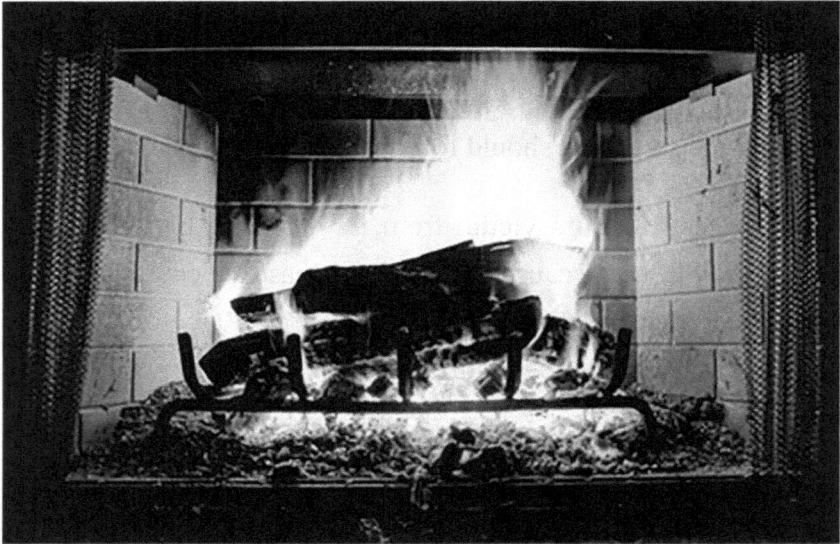

Minor Burns

These are the steps you should follow for first-degree and second-degree burns.

1. Start by holding the burnt area under some cool running water. Note, this water should not be cold. An alternative could be applying a wet compress on the area until the pain goes down.

2. Ensure you remove any tight items or rings from the area that's burnt quickly but gently before swelling starts.

3. Ensure you don't break any blisters. The fluid-filled ones are great at protecting against infections. If the blister somehow ends up breaking, you should clean the area with some water and mild soap. The soap is optional, though. You should then apply an antibiotic ointment, but in case it causes rashes, discontinue use.

4. Apply some lotion to the burn once it is cooled completely. If you can find one with aloe vera, that would be great. The lotion will help the area from drying up and offers relief to the burn victim.

5. Tie a bandage around the burn. Ensure you wrap it loosely to avoid causing pressure on the burnt area as this could be painful. Bandaging, aside from reducing pain, keeps air off the area and protects the area of the skin that's blistered.

6. You can give the burn victim over-the-counter medication which could include ibuprofen, naproxen sodium or acetaminophen.

REMEMBER: If you're in a life-threatening or emergency medical situation, seek medical assistance immediately.

Chapter 5

Choking and Basic First Aid

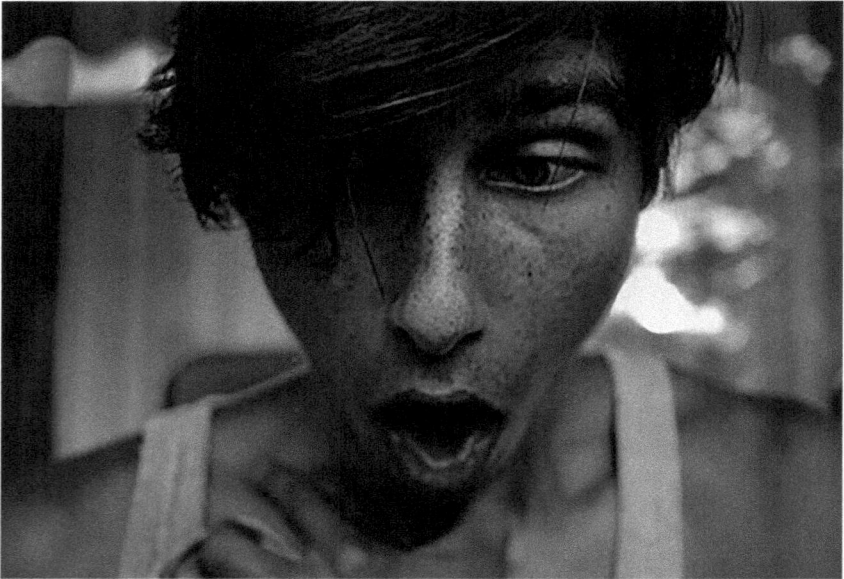

Signs from Choking

• Hand signals. The first thing a person who is choking will do is to try and send you a signal, often with their hands. This is because they are unable to talk. They could panic and start to wave as a way of asking for help.

- Inability to breathe properly. If you look at someone and notice that they are struggling to breathe, it could be that they are choking. The victim could start wheezing, gagging, or coughing. If the object has completely blocked the victim's airway, they might be completely unable to breathe. In case it's an infant, they could have a weak cough or go completely quiet.

- Clutching of the throat. This, just like hand signals, is a very natural reaction by choking victims and the easiest for a person to notice.

- Blue lips and skin. Usually, a choking victim will be suffocating, so it's common for their faces, lips, or fingertips if not all of these to turn blue. This is because they are unable to get sufficient oxygen to their blood. This is a sign that might not appear immediately because it normally takes some time for the amount of oxygen in the blood to reduce, so it's worth being very alert and aware of the other symptoms.

- The victim could pass out because of a lack of oxygen in the brain. If you notice that a victim's chest has stopped rising and falling or if you suddenly cannot hear them breathing, you should immediately unblock their airway

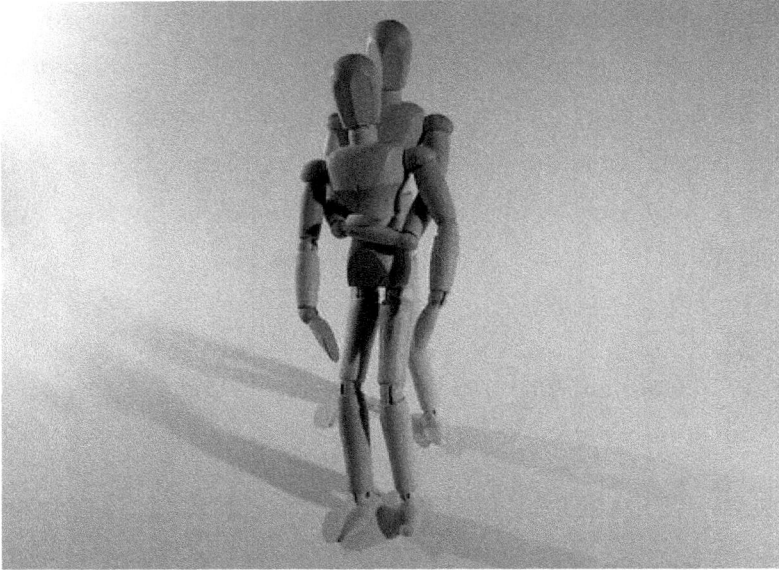

First Aid for Choking Accidents

In case the choking victim can cough forcefully, make sure they keep coughing. If they can't, then you could start the first aid process by:

1. Giving the victim five back blows. Stand beside the choking victim, just right behind them if they are an adult. If they're a child, kneel down behind them. You should then place your arm around the victim's chest to give them support. Bend the victim over at their waist to ensure the upper part of their body is parallel with the floor or ground. Give the victim five back blows separately between their shoulder blades using the heel of your hand

2. Give the victim five abdominal thrusts which are called the Heimlich maneuver.

3. Alternate between the blows and the thrusts until you manage to dislodge the blockage

In order for you to perform abdominal thrusts on someone else do the following:

1. Stand behind them with one foot slightly ahead of the other so that you have balance. Wrap your hands around the victim's waist then slightly tip them forward. If it's a child, kneel behind them.

2. With one of your hands, make a fist and position it above the victim's navel.

3. With your other hand, grasp the fist and press it hard into the victim's abdomen with a fast upward thrust.

4. Do the thrusts six to ten times until you manage to dislodge the blockage. In case you're the only one administering first aid, ensure you perform both backflows and abdominal thrusts before you call for emergency help. If there's someone else with you, have them call for help while you perform first aid on the victim.

If the victim is unconscious, perform cardiopulmonary resuscitation with rescue breaths and chest compressions.

In case you're performing abdominal thrusts on yourself, try as much as possible to call for emergency help. Although it will be difficult, try to deliver abdominal thrusts to ensure the item is dislodged. To do so:

1. Place one of your fists above the navel.

2. Use the other hand to grasp your fist and bend over a countertop, chair or any other hard surface.

3. Shove your fist both inwards and upwards.

In case you're clearing a pregnant woman's airway or that of an obese person:

- Place your hands a bit higher than you would on a different person, at the breastbone base. The position just above where the lowest ribs join.

- Press hard into the victim's chest giving a quick thrust.

- Repeat this process until food, or the cause of blockage is dislodged.

- In case the person loses consciousness from choking, you can proceed as follows to clear their airway:

- Lower them on their back onto the floor ensuring their arms are on the side.

- In case the cause of blockage is visible at the back of the victim's throat, or maybe if it's high in their throat, put your finger in their mouth and sweep it out. Note that you should not try a finger sweep if you can't see the blockage object as this could push the finger deep into the victim's airway. This can happen very easily in younger children.

- Start CPR in case the object stays lodged and if there's no response from the victim after you've taken these measures. The chest compressions that you'll use while you do the CPR could help dislodge the object. Recheck the victim's mouth periodically.

If you're clearing the airway of a child who's below a year old, follow the procedure below:

- Sit and hold the infant that's choking face down on your forearm that should be resting on your thigh. Use your hand to support their head and neck and then place their head lower than the trunk.

- Proceed to thump the infant firmly but ensure you do it gently about five times. Do it in the middle of their back using your hand's heel. The back blows combined with gravity should release the object that's choking them. Ensure your fingers remain pointed up so that you don't hit the infant at the back of their head.

- Turn the infant so that they are faceup on your forearm. You should have them resting on your thigh with their head lower than the trunk, that's if the infant is still not breathing. Place two fingers at the center of the choking infant's breastbone and compress the chest five times. Do it quickly. If you're wondering how far down you should press, 1 ½ inch will be great and then allow the chest to rise again between the compressions.

- Keep repeating the chest thrusts and the back blows call 911.

- In case none of these steps work for the choking infant breathing but it does opens the airway, start CPR to help them breathe.

Chapter 6

Falls and Basic First Aid

First Aid for Domestic Falls

In case someone falls at home, you can do the following as part of first aid so that they feel better faster:

1. If the person has lost consciousness, run through the ABC of the basic first aid. In case the person isn't breathing, or the person's heart isn't beating, apply CPR.

2. Clean any visible wounds with water. It's preferred to clean open wounds with distilled water, but running water can suffice as long as it's clean.

3. Grab an ice pack and apply it to the injury area so that any swelling or pain can be reduced. When you're doing this, ensure the ice is not directly on the victim's skin, so it's better to wrap the ice pack with a clean towel.

4. In case there is any bleeding stop it by applying some pressure using a clean piece of cloth and a sterile dressing. Sterile gauze bandages are preferred to apply pressure over

bleeding wounds, to prevent contamination and infections from happening.

5. Fractured bones are very common in falls, so it's important to avoid moving the person too much until there's a certainty that there aren't any broken bones. If there are any fractures, place the necessary immobilizations. More information about diagnosing a broken bone and what to do with them can be found in chapter twelve.

6. Do your best to comfort the individual and if you can, find out the details of the fall.

7. In case you do not see any injuries, advise the fall victim to rest for some time before you help them stand up slowly.

8. In case the fall victim is an elderly person, monitor them closely for a day or two to ensure there are no other symptoms that could be dangerous to their overall health.

9. In case the victim has an open cut from the fall, you should ensure they get a tetanus shot.

10. You can have the victim take an over-the-counter painkiller if they are experiencing pain.

11. If the pain is persistent, they are confused, unable to walk or move any body parts, then seek emergency help professional assessment.

Remember, you should always call an ambulance if:

- There is heavy bleeding on the area they landed on or if the blood is coming from their nose, mouth or ears.

- If you suspect the victim has suffered an injury on their neck, back, or their hip. Failure to get emergency help for this could actually cause further complications that could be permanent or even worse, fatal.

- If the fall victim is having a hard time breathing.

- If the fall victim is unconscious or unable to move.

Chapter 7

Poisoning, Overdose, and Basic First Aid

Poison Control Center

1-800-822-1222

Or

www.poison.org

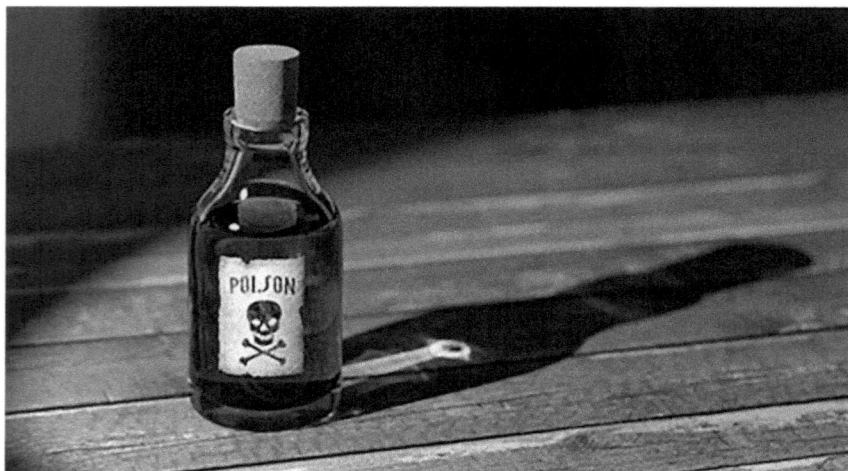

Symptoms of Poisoning and Overdose

Poisoning and overdose symptoms are highly dependent on the type of substance taken and the amount. Some of the general symptoms include:

- A feeling of general sickness

- Diarrhea

- Stomach pains, sometimes very sharp

- Dizziness or drowsiness

- Pupils can be dilated

- They can feel weak

- Increase body temperature

- Shivering and body chills

- Slight or severe headaches

- They can be irritable

- Difficulty breathing / shortness of breath

- It can be hard for the patient to swallow

- They can produce more saliva than usual or have foaming of the mouth

- Skin rashes

- Blue lips and skin

- Burns around their mouth and nose

- Blurred vision

- Mental confusion with or without slurred speech

- Seizures

- They can lose consciousness

- The patient can fall into a coma

Aspirin Overdose

Specific symptoms include:

- Sweating

- Increased respiratory rate

- The victim can experience ringing in their ears

- Temporary loss of hearing

Tricyclic Antidepressants Overdose

Specific symptoms include:

- Excitability

- Severe dry mouth

- Enlarged pupils

- Rapid or irregular heartbeat

- Low blood pressure and the victim could become lightheaded

Serotonin Reuptake Inhibitors (SSRIs) Overdose

These are specific type of antidepressant such as Paxil, Zoloft, Prozac, etc.

Specific symptoms include:

- Agitation

- Victims eyes could move uncontrollably

- They may experience severe tension in their muscles

Beta-Blocker and Calcium Channel Blocker Overdose

Beta-blockers are used in the treatment of heart and blood conditions. Signs of an overdose include:

- Low blood pressure which can cause lightheadedness and fainting

- A slow heart rate

- A feeling of agitation

- Chest pain

Benzodiazepine Overdose

Common drugs include Xanax, Diazepam, Valium, etc.

The specific signs of overdose can include:

- Poor coordination and difficulty in speech

- Uncontrollable eye movement

- Shallow breathing

- Episodes of drowsiness

Opioid Overdose

Common examples include Morphine, Hydrocodone, Heroine, etc.

Signs to look out for include:

- A reduction in the size of the victim's pupils

- Shallow breathing

- Drowsiness

- Loss of consciousness

- Needle marks from drug injection

Stimulant Overdose

Symptoms including:

- Hallucinations

1. Restless or agitated

2. Chest pains

3. Increased body temperature

4. Rapid breathing

5. Irregular or fast heartbeat

First Aid for Poisoning

The kind of first aid offered to poison victims is dependent on the victim's symptoms, age, and the amount of substance that caused poisoning. There's need to call for help if you notice the victim is experiencing the following symptoms:

- Drowsiness or if the victim is unconscious

- If the victim is having trouble breathing or even worse if they've stopped breathing altogether

- If the poisoning victim is uncontrollably agitated or appears very restless

- If the victim is also experiencing seizures

- If the victim is on some kind of medication or any other kind of substance and accidentally or intentionally overdosed

The first aid steps you could take to help the poisoning victim include:

1. For swallowed poison, you could start by removing anything that's left in the victim's mouth. In case the source of poisoning is a cleaning agent, acid, or any other product that comes packaged, check the label for instructions in case of poisoning. Call the poison control center. 1-800-822-1222

2. When the poison is in the victim's eyes, remember that every second is crucial; otherwise, they could end up blind. If they have contact lenses, remove them and use plenty of water that's at room temperature to irrigate the eye for between fifteen to twenty minutes. If the victim is either an adult or an older child, they could simply hop into a shower for this. However, if they're a younger child, wrap them in a towel and use the faucet in your kitchen sink to irrigate their eyes. Another alternative is to pour water using a pitcher. Ensure the water is hitting the bridge of the nose and avoid pouring it directly into the eye. After irrigating the eye, let it rest and then call for help, preferably from poison control. If, after an hour, the victim still feels some irritation or pain or if they experience redness, some visual problems or swelling, they will need to get an ophthalmic exam urgently. This will require a trip to the emergency room. If in doubt, call 911.

3. If the victim inhaled the poison, quickly move them to an area with fresh air. Keep them away from any toxic fumes and ensure the area is thoroughly ventilated. If they are experiencing difficulty breathing, seek emergency medical treatment.

4. When the poison is on the skin, put on gloves and remove any contaminated clothing, then thoroughly rinse the skin for fifteen minutes in a shower or using a hose. For this, every second count, so do your best to avoid any delays. Make sure the water is at room temperature, and you could use some mild soap to eliminate any material that remains stuck to the skin. Call poison control if you're unsure. After this, you could seek further instructions from a medical practitioner, or take the victim to the emergency room.

5. When you're getting emergency assistance, ensure you gather any bottles of possible causes of the poisoning to give to the emergency personnel.

REMEMBER: If you're in a life-threatening or emergency medical situation, seek medical assistance immediately.

Chapter 8

Near Drowning and Basic First Aid

Symptoms from Near-Drowning

- The victim's skin could turn bluish and become very cold

- There could be swelling in the abdomen

- The victim could experience some pain around their chest area

- The victim could also cough continuously

- It's common for the near-drowning victim to have shortness of breath

- There could be vomiting because the victim probably drank a lot of the water unintentionally during the unpleasant experience

- The near-drowning victim could be irritable for a while or show other unusual behavior

- A lack of energy after the water incident. The victim could feel extremely tired

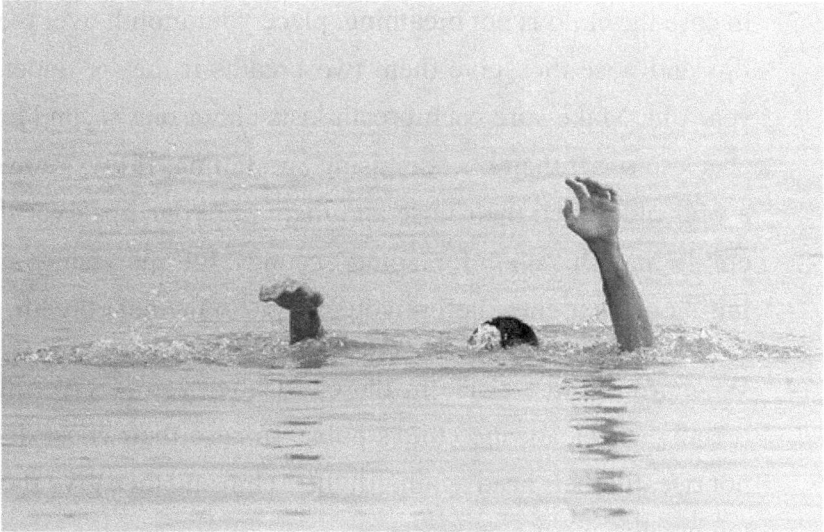

First Aid for Near-Drowning

When your child has a near-drowning experience, you can offer first aid through:

1. Getting them out of the water quickly. This is the first priority because when you fail to do so, they could actually end up drowning. In case the child is not breathing you should place them on their back on a surface that's firm then begin rescue breathing as you have someone else help you in calling for help.

2. Open the child's airway by gently tilting their head back using one hand. Lift the child's chin using the other hand. Place

your ear on both the child's mouth and their nose. Check, listen, and try to feel for any signs that the child is breathing.

3. In case the child is not breathing, place your mouth over their lips and nose then give them two breaths if they're under a year old. Make sure each breath lasts about one second and check to see if their chest is rising and falling. If they're over a year old, pinch their nose and then seal your lips over the child's mouth. Wait for some seconds for the rising and falling of their chest before you give them the next breath.

4. When you notice a rise in the chest after you've given the breaths, check for the child's pulse. In case their chest does not rise, tilt their head again, lift their chin and then give them the breaths again.

5. Use two fingers on the victim's neck to the side of their Adam's apple to check for a pulse. If the child is still an infant, you can check for a pulse by feeling inside their arm between their elbow and shoulder then wait for about five seconds. In case the child does have a pulse, make sure you give them a breath every three seconds and keep checking for a pulse after every one minute. You should keep on rescue breathing until the victim can breathe on their own.

6. In case you cannot find a pulse, place two fingers between the chest of the child if they're under a year old and apply chest compressions. Doing five-inch ones in about three seconds will help to a great extent. After this, place your lips

over the child's nose and mouth and give them one breath. If the victim is above a year old, use the heel of your hand and apply one-inch chest compressions in the middle of their breastbone. Do about five of them quickly, after which you should pinch the child's nose, then place your lips over their mouth then give them a full breath.

7. You need to keep on giving the chest compressions, and the breaths until you find a pulse or paramedics arrive.

8. When a child has had a near-drowning experience and appears unresponsive, never assume it's too late to save their life. Keep performing CPR on them until help arrives.

REMEMBER: If you're in a life-threatening or emergency medical situation, seek medical assistance immediately.

Chapter 9

Sprains and Basic First Aid

First Aid for Sprains

The most common types of sprains are ankle sprains. However, you could also experience sprains on your wrists, thumb, and knees. Whenever you have a sprained ligament, you will experience pain and rapid swelling. The more the pain and the greater the swelling, the more severe the injury. For minor injuries, you can do some first aid, through the RICE formula that is:

1. Rest- Ensure the injured limb is well-rested. It's often recommended that you avoid placing anything heavy on the limb for between forty-eight to seventy-two hours. You might actually need to use crutches. In some cases, a brace or a splint could come in handy, especially in the initial stages. However, make sure you don't completely avoid all activity. Even if the sprain is on your ankle, you should always move around and exercise, as this reduces the deconditioning.

2. Ice- Grab a cold pack or a compression sleeve full of cold water and use it on the sprain to prevent further swelling.

After this, put some ice on the area for about fifteen to twenty minutes. It will be even more helpful to do it within the first two days or up until you notice a significant reduction in swelling. Keep the ice for a reasonable period, as having it there for a very long time will lead to tissue damage.

3. Compress- Use a bandage to compress the area. You could also use an elastic wrap.

4. Elevate- Keep the sprained area elevated. A position above your heart will either help or reduce swelling.

It could take several days or even months for a sprain to heal, but as you notice or experience a reduction in the swelling or pain, you can slowly start moving the injured area. While it's still painful, you could take some over-the-counter painkillers such as ibuprofen, acetaminophen, among others. Before you fully go back to activities like sports or working out, it's very important to restore the strength of the injured area. You could even consider seeking the services of a physical therapist to help you exercise the area so that you do not end up injuring it further.

You should seek medical advice if your sprain fails to improve after three days. If you get a sprain, you might need emergency assistance if:

- You can't bear having some weight on the injured area. You should also do so if the area is numb, feels unstable, or in case you can't use that particular joint. If you're experiencing this, it could be that your ligament got completely torn.

- In case you notice some redness around the sprained area or if you can see some red streaks spreading out of the injured area. This is a sign of infection.

- If you experience some pain over that area of the sprain

- If you've ended up injuring an area that's been strained a couple of times in the past

- If the sprain appears to be very severe because when you delay treatment for this, it could lead to instability and cause chronic pain

Chapter 10

Bruises, Abrasions and Basic First Aid

Soft Tissue Damage

It's very difficult to diagnose this, but when you have soft tissue damage, you could experience a lot of pain. These injuries are usually not visible, but you will feel some soreness in your body, and sometimes this could happen days after the domestic fall. If left untreated, these injuries could cause chronic pain and could even worse, lead to other injuries or pain in other body parts because you overuse these other parts to compensate for the pain.

First Aid for Bruises

In case someone has a bruise at home, you could solve it in the following ways:

1. Rest- Ensure that the specific area that's bruised is well-rested before you proceed

2. Ice-Grab an ice pack and wrap it in a towel then place it on the bruise. Leave it there for between ten to twenty minutes.

Ensure you do this several times within the day for about two days or as is needed

3. Compress- Compress the area in case it's starting to swell. Use an elastic bandage for this but make sure you don't tighten it too much

4. Elevate- Keep the bruised part elevated

If the victim's skin is not broken, then you will not need to use a bandage. You could just have them take some painkillers for any pain they could be experiencing.

These steps should help, but in case you notice the following, you should seek further medical advice:

- Some painful swelling in the area around the bruise

- If the pain persists after three days despite the injury seeming minor

- If you keep getting frequent bruises especially on the back or face area and on the trunk

- If you notice that you get bruises easily and perhaps have a history of bleeding that was because of a surgical procedure

- If you notice a lump occurring on the bruise

- If you seem to be bleeding abnormally, especially from your nose or the gums

- If you have a family history of bleeding or bruising easily

Chapter 11

Head Injuries and Basic First Aid

Symptoms of a Head Injury

You should also look out for any head injuries when you fall at home. Many people who are victims of a domestic fall will feel a mild headache if they hit their head and often think it's nothing to worry about. However, you should be concerned and, if possible, get to a medical facility as soon as possible so that you have some tests done just to be sure. If you hit your head, look out for symptoms such as:

- Loss of balance

- Sudden headaches or intense ones that keep growing worse

- Nausea

- Dizziness

- Listlessness

- Changes in the level of consciousness (sleepiness).

- Confusion

- Trouble speaking

- Seizures

- Incapacity or weakness to use a limb.

- Blood or fluids leaking through the nose and/or ears.

- Severe facial or head bleeding.

- Additional signs in children may include persistent crying, repeated vomiting, bulging in the head's soft spot, and refusal to eat.

First Aid for Head Injury

A non-trained person can't assess the possible dangerous complications of a head injury, especially since that requires medical equipment. All head injuries must be evaluated by a physician to make sure there aren't internal consequences hidden from the naked eye.

If the head injury is so severe that it creates an open wound (skin rupture and bleeding), or there are signs of severity, here are the steps you should follow:

1. Immediately call for medical assistance – call 911: Until the paramedics arrive at the scene, it's best to avoid moving the person as much as possible to retain from worsening any possible spinal injuries.

2. Stop bleeding: If there's bleeding coming from an open wound, use a sterile gauze bandage or a clean cloth to apply pressure over the wound and stop the bleeding. If there are reasons to believe that the skull may be fractured, the direct pressure can't be applied. Don't stop bleeding or fluid leakage through the nose or ears; if possible, tilt the head forward to allow the fluid to exit through the nose instead of going through the opposite way and falling towards the pharynx, esophagus, and ultimately stomach.

3. Initiate CPR to resume breathing and heartbeats if they stop: Persons with severe head trauma may have an interruption in the body's vital functions depending on the affected area of the brain. Be aware of any changes in the heart rate or respiratory rate and react accordingly, following the CPR instructions described in the first chapter.

REMEMBER: If you're in a life-threatening or emergency medical situation, seek medical assistance immediately.

Chapter 12

Broken Bones and Basic First Aid

Symptoms

If you have someone in front of you that fell from a tree, rolled down a hill, or had any other form of a traumatic accident, the first thing you must do before you attempt to move this person is to identify whether there's a fractured bone or not. Here are the signs you must look for in fractures:

- Pain: A fractured bone is going to hurt very much, especially with movement.

- Functional incapacity: Body segments with broken bones can't move, and they're often unable to support the weight. So, a broken leg won't be able to move, and the person won't be able to step over it without falling down.

- Swelling or bruising: The affected body segment will increase in volume, and often will turn reddish, purple, or pale depending on the consequences of the broken bone.

- Deformation: Fractures will change the shape of the affected body segment depending on their severity.

- Open fracture: Sometimes the fractured bone will make itself evident by protruding out of the wound and making itself visible.

Remember that fractures aren't always developed after a traumatic event; sometimes bones can be fractured in the daily routine, for no apparent reason. So you must think about fractures whenever you see these symptoms even if there wasn't a traumatic event.

Some other conditions such as muscle sprains and dislocations are very similar to fractures, and they're treated the same way in first aid, so if you're confused about whether you have a dislocated bone, a broken bone, or a strained muscle, the first aid will be the same.

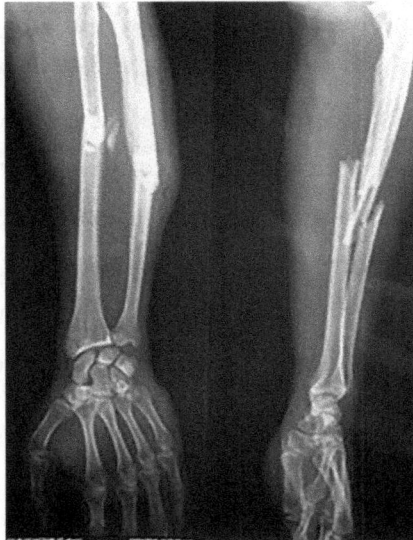

First Aid for Broken Bones

First aid for broken bones spins around immobilizing them. Fractures tend to get worse with movement, and they'll always need professional medical assistance to heal, so your job in first aid is to call for the emergency service and immobilize the person until the paramedics arrive at the scene. In the worst-case scenario, you'll have to immobilize the person until it's safe to take the person to an emergency service in a trauma center or hospital.

Rules for Immobilization

There are three main rules you should follow with any immobilizations.

- **Look for stability:** Always use something strong and able to adapt to the shape of the body's segment to keep the fractured bone in a stable position. Commercial splints and cervical collars are preferred for this, so it's highly advisable to have them available. If there aren't any commercial splints available, it's acceptable and necessary to create improvised splints. Planks, sticks, shoes, cardboard, anything adaptable to the body and strong enough to keep it stable can make an acceptable splint. Use bandages to set the improvised immobilizations in place; if there are no bandages available, strings, belts, and even shoelaces can be used in their place.

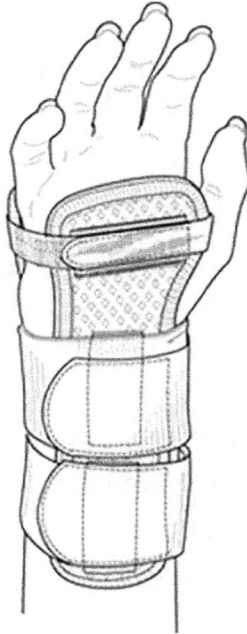

- **Secure the joints:** Fractured bones of the limbs should always be immobilized securing the proximal and distal joints; these are, the joint that's further from the body, and the joint that's closer to the body. Using a fractured forearm as an example, you should always immobilize the wrist (distal joint) and the elbow (proximal joint) to prevent the fractured bone from moving. With a fractured thigh, you should always immobilize the knee (distal joint) and the hip (proximal joint).

- **Allow blood and airflow:** A common amateur mistake is to tie the splint so hard towards the affected body segment that the blood flow is interrupted. This is a dangerous situation that's only acceptable when trying to apply a tourniquet to stop massive bleeding from a limb. If an immobilized limb turns pale or blue, this tells us that there may be a blood-flow interruption, and the splint must be loosened. In the case of cervical immobilizations, pale or blue skin color in the face could either mean blood-flow or air-flow interruption; both of these situations are extremely dangerous and must be dealt with immediately. Once again, the immobilization must be loosened.

A quick way to make sure that the circulation isn't compromised is to feel the pulse of the immobilized limb. It's standard procedure to feel the pulse of the limb once the immobilization has been placed, and to loosen up the straps or the bandages if there's no perceivable pulse.

Immobilizations According to the Affected Body Segment

There are specific immobilization techniques that depend on the fractured bone.

- **Cervical spine immobilization:** This is the first immobilization that should be applied to polytraumatized persons because cervical spine injuries carry the worst complications out of all fractures. The best way to do a cervical spine immobilization is by using a cervical collar. If you don't have a cervical collar available, you can use a pair of hats, a pair of shoes, cardboard, pillows, or anything able to keep the neck from rotating or tilting to either side.

It's important to keep the neck in a stable position while applying the immobilization, so it's best to do it with the help of another person. One person is in charge of lifting the person by the neck and the back, keeping the neck in a fixed position, while the other second sets the immobilization in place. Then, the person is laid once more over the surface and the immobilization is strapped in place. Remember to check that the blood-flow and air-flow aren't compromised.

- **Arm immobilizations:** These are the most common immobilizations due to the frequency of arm fractures. Arm immobilizations are done with splints and slings.

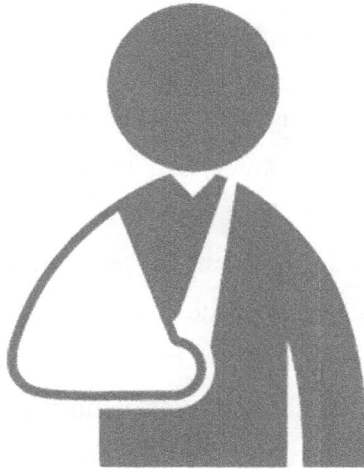

Splinting is the first step for arm immobilizations. Among splints, commercial splints are preferred, but if there aren't any available, feel free to use planks, sticks, cardboard, or anything else that may be adapted to the neck. The right position to immobilize the arm is by bending the elbow in a ninety degrees angle, sometimes an even closer angle for lower arm injuries (forearm, wrist, and hand).

Remember to follow the second rule for immobilizations and remain from moving proximal and distal joints.

A sling will be your next step once you've placed a splint. Slings are done to secure the splinted arm to the body, avoiding any movements. It's better to do arm slings with triangular bandages. If there are no triangular bandages, pieces of cloth that could be bent as triangular bandages are also acceptable. However, if this isn't possible either, regular pressure bandages or even belts can also be used. Slings can also help control a bleeding arm by elevating it. There are three main sling techniques that you must dominate; two of them need a triangular bandage, and the other one fulfills their purpose if no triangular bandage is available.

First you have the arm sling, the most common type of sling. This is fit for immobilizing the upper arm (shoulder, humerus, rib, and clavicle immobilization). You start the arm sling by placing the triangular bandage under the arm, the point of the bandage pointing at the elbow, the longer side of the bandage facing in the direction of the feet, and the shorter side of the bandage towards the healthy shoulder. Then, the top side is taken behind the neck, towards the bandaged shoulder. Next, the longer side is taken up, over the patient's forearm, and in the direction of the injured shoulder towards the other tip of the bandage. Tie the tips of the bandage together and tuck the corners of the know below the bandage for comfort. The arm must be placed horizontally, with only a slight elevation towards the affected arm. The sling is finally done by extending the fabric towards the fingertips. It's helpful to tie the fabric behind and below the elbow to improve arm stability.

Next you have the elevated arm sling. This is the other sling that requires a triangular bandage, and it's fit for lower arm fractures and injuries (hand, wrist, and forearm). It's great to stop bleeding in this area because of the elevation. However, remember the second rule of immobilizations. If the elbow isn't already in a bent position, then it's better not to use it if you suspect a fracture. The first step is to place the arm diagonally over the chest, hand aimed at the healthy shoulder. The second step is to place the triangular bandage over the arm with one end over the healthy shoulder and the point towards the elbow. Then, the lower edge of the bandage must be carefully tucked under the forearm and elbow. The fourth step is to take the free end of the bandage behind the patient's back and diagonally towards the healthy shoulder, where it's tied to the other end. Finally, the corners of the knot are tucked under and the piece of fabric behind the elbow is tied to improve stability and comfort.

If there's nothing like a triangular bandage available, the best option is to use a collar-and-cuff sling. This only needs a compression bandage, but a belt, a string, or anything else that may be adapted as a compression bandage can be used. This sling also allows a varying degree of flexion for the elbow, so it's ideal for fractured persons that need the arm in a flexion wider than 90 degrees. It begins by placing the center of the bandage behind the person's neck and healthy shoulder, with the two ends falling at both sides. Then, the arm must be placed in the desired position, with the intended flexion of the elbow (if you suspect a fracture, the arm should be left the way you found it). The sling is done once you tie both ends of the bandage around the patient's wrist, tying a knot below it.

- **Leg immobilizations:** Commercial splints come prepared to immobilize the leg in the right position, but if there are no commercial splints available, learning to immobilize a leg is still an easy task. The leg is much easier to immobilize than the arms because of the preferred position to secure it. It has to be immobilized with only a small flexion of the knee; this slight flexion can be achieved by placing a roll of bandage under the knee. Then, the whole leg is immobilized by securing it against a hard and long object able to adapt to its shape and stabilize it. Planks, long sticks, and even cardboard can be used as a splint, secured by compression bandages, belts, or anything available to tie the splint. If there are no suitable objects available, it's acceptable to tie the injured leg to the healthy leg, using the healthy leg as a splint.

- **Back immobilizations:** Thoracic spine and lumbar spine are also very vulnerable to fractures, and these fractures are dangerous for their terrible consequences. However, the only way to properly immobilize the thoracic and lumbar spine is with a stretcher, and it's a delicate procedure that must be taken care of by health professionals. So, if you suspect thoracic and/or lumbar spine fracture, the best course of action is to try to immobilize the cervical spine without tilting or rotating the back, and call professional help to come to the person's aid. The only situation in which you should try to mobilize someone with a suspected thoracic and/or lumbar fracture is when there's no professional help available, and you need to transport the person to a hospital on your own. In this particular case, the best way to do it is by carrying the person with the help of three other persons. Two at either side must be holding the torso in place, one must be holding the head and taking care of the neck, and the last one must be carrying the legs and keeping them straight. This is the safest way to carry someone with a suspected broken back without a stretcher; however, it's still better to wait for professional help.

Chapter 13

Stokes and Basic First Aid

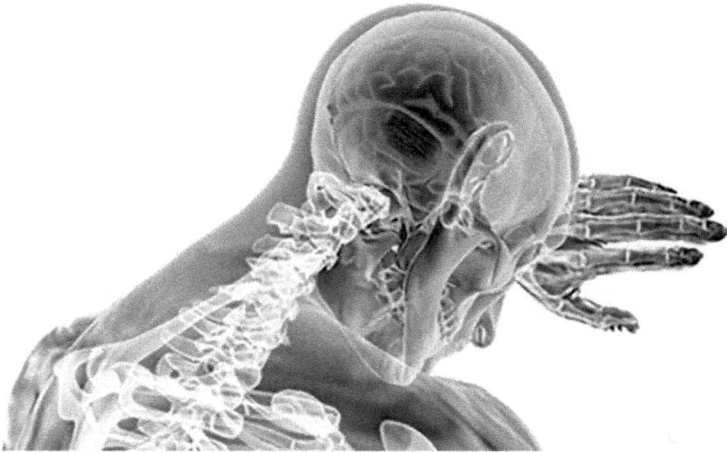

Symptoms

The symptoms of a stroke depend on the affected area of the brain and they can take on a wide range of neurological manifestations. Strokes are a medical emergency. Symptoms can include:

- Headache.

- Paralysis of one side of the body (or both sides).

- Paralysis of one side (or both sides) of the face.

- Slurred speech.

- Trouble walking.

- Sensitive impairments (on one side or both sides of the body).

- Hallucinations.

- Seizures.

- Muscular weakness (either localized, to a side, or general).

Whenever you suspect there's a stroke developing in a person, you should follow a four-step route to identify it quickly and act upon it. This four-step route goes by the acronym of "F.A.S.T":

- Face: Ask the person to smile. If the person's facial expression is asymmetrical, this is a sign of facial paralysis, that's a common manifestation of a stroke.

- Arms: Ask the person to raise both arms at the same height. If one arm is lower than the other, or unable to ascend at all, this is a sign of paralysis, another common manifestation of a stroke.

- Speech: Ask the person to say a simple phrase. If the person has trouble speaking, or is unable to speak, this is a sign of a stroke. Also, a general incapacity to understand when spoken to is another sign of a stroke.

- Time: If any of these signs are identified, it's time to call 911.

First Aid for Strokes

Strokes are severe medical conditions that need to be acted upon immediately. When a stroke is identified, the person must receive medical assistance immediately. In the meantime, these are the general steps you should follow, the only things that can be done with a stroke as first aid.

- Don't provide medication: Strokes are extremely delicate conditions and they should be left for the medical professionals. Don't provide any sort of medication; if the person is consuming alcohol and any other form of legal or illegal drug, stop its consumption immediately.

- Avoid moving the person: If the person fell and received trauma to the head, treat the injury as possible spinal harm and act accordingly with immobilizations (as described in the previous chapter).

- Safe position: The person should be placed in a comfortable position, with the head slightly elevated and the body moved to a side to be prepared for vomiting.

- Keep temperature: Keep the person warm using a blanket or anything else available.

- Monitor the condition: Keep track of the person's heart rate and respiratory rate. If the person ever stops breathing, or the heart stops beating, provide respiratory CPR or CPR immediately.

Chapter 14

Heart Attacks and Basic First Aid

Symptoms

A heart attack is an acute syndrome that manifests powerfully. The person will experience pain in the chest, along with a feeling of aching, tightness, pressure, and/or squeezing sensation that can also be felt in the left arm, the left side of the neck, and the left side of the jaw. Heart attacks are a medical emergency. Other symptoms associated with a heart attack are:

- Abdominal pain or nausea.

- Coughing.

- Vomiting.

- Shortness of breath.

- Fatigue.

- Cold sweat.

- A general feeling of terror.

The symptoms may vary depending on the person and the severity of the heart attack. Severe heart attacks will hurt much more than lesser heart attacks; however, all heart attacks are relevant and people suffering a heart attack should always be taken to a hospital as soon as possible.

First Aid for Heart Attacks

In the case of a heart attack, there's no risk in taking care of the person's transportation to the hospital. However, there's an invaluable service provided by ambulances that greatly increases the survival rate of the patients they transport, and it's that they keep close communication with the hospitals to let them know they're going there with a critical patient, preparing them before the patient arrives. So, don't take the patient to a hospital yourself unless you're certain that the ambulance will take too long and you're able to transport the patient much faster. In the meantime, here are the basic steps you should follow as first aid for a possible heart attack:

- Take an aspirin: Aspirins are the first step to treat a heart attack, and they're the only medicine that can be provided safely without medical supervision. Swallowing an aspirin, or even chewing it and swallowing it, will help the person dissolve the blood clot that's probably obstructing the coronary artery.

- Comfortable position: Take the person to a seated position, allowing the person some breathing space to relax.

- CPR: In heart attacks you must be on the lookout for cardiorespiratory arrest. So, if the person's heart stops beating, start Cardiopulmonary Resuscitation immediately until help arrives.

Chapter 15

Suffocation and Basic First Aid

S uffocation isn't a singular disease, but several different diseases involved with an interruption of the supply of oxygen to the body. Suffocation through being submerged in a large body of water (drowning) has already been covered in the eight chapters, so here we'll cover the general instances of oxygen deprivation and shortness of breath.

Symptoms

These are the general symptoms of lack of oxygen:

- Increased respiratory rate.

- Feeling of suffocation.

- Pale face.

- Blue or purple lips and fingernails.

- Feeling tired, dizzy, or faint.

First Aid for Suffocation

The first-aid approach to treat suffocation can get as diverse as the different causes behind it.

General Measures

If no underlying critical conditions are causing the suffocation, such as heart attacks, asthma attacks, or important bleedings, there are many things to do that could alleviate the suffocation symptoms while medical help is contacted.

- Tilt the person's torso forward.

- Allow some breathing room to the person.

- Use fans or any means necessary to blow air towards the person.

- Make sure the airways of the person aren't obstructed or compromised in any way.

- If the person isn't breathing, start Respiratory CPR as soon as possible (as described in the first chapter of this book).

Infant Suffocation

In case you suspect infant suffocation or strangulation (air deprivation through external compression of the airways, often due to a cable or chord), no matter how long the infant may have been deprived of oxygen, these are the general steps to follow:

- Remove the harming object: Take away the pillow or sheets that may have been suffocating the infant as soon as possible. In the case of strangulation, sometimes it may be easier to use scissors to remove the constricting object.

- Check vital signs: Check if the infant is breathing and the heart is beating. If not, start CPR immediately.

The technique for CPR on infants is very similar to the technique for CPR in adults. However, there are a couple of differences that need to be noted.

It's no longer necessary to close the nose while blowing air through the mouth for the rescue breaths. Instead, the mouth seal should cover both the mouth and the nose of the infant. Don't blow as hard as you would if you were performing CPR on an adult, and make sure to check that the infant's abdomen isn't raising with the rescue breaths.

Regarding the chest compressions, you should use two fingers to compress the infant's sternum instead of using two hands. The chest must be lowered about 1.5 inches deep, and no more than that.

Other than that, there are no differences. CPR must continue until breathing resumes or professional help arrives at the scene.

Specific Measures

Whenever you see an adult that's suffocating for no apparent reason, you must consider any medical disease that the person may be suffering and act accordingly. Medical conditions that could cause suffocation symptoms include:

- Asthma attacks: This person probably knows about the asthma diagnosis, so the diagnosis is straightforward.

- Heart attack: Search for the typical chest pain of a heart attack.

- Respiratory infections: This person is probably sick. The symptoms of respiratory infections include fever, cough, and congestion.

- Sudden blood loss: Look for wounds or bruises that may signal internal bleeding.

Chapter 16

Home Remedies for Domestic Accidents

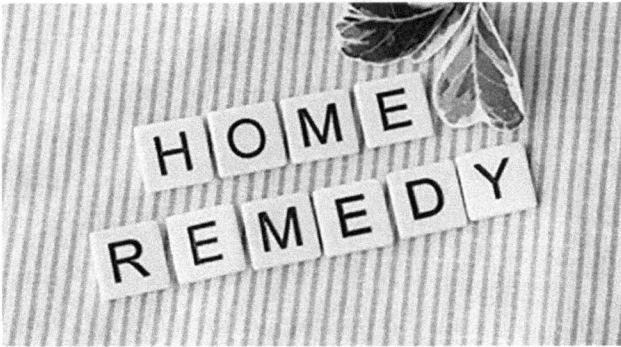

What are Home Remedies?

Home remedies refer to medication that's prepared and administered without the prescription of a doctor or generally without professional supervision.

Benefits of Using Home Remedies for Domestic Accidents

If you've injured yourself at home and can't get prescription medication or if they don't seem to be working as well as you'd like them to, you could try natural home remedies instead. Home remedies can be used for different injuries. They are very inexpensive as they often involve things we already have. Here are more reasons why you should consider home remedies:

Home Remedies Help You Heal Your Injuries Naturally

Normally, prescription medication is mostly synthetic. These kinds of medications contain substances that are not good for your body. While they could help with solving the problem of an injury, they could cause another problem in a different body organ. They could trigger some allergies or breathing difficulties and could leave you with some side effects. Natural home remedies, on the other hand, support the ability of your body to heal itself. While they heal your injury, they also boost your immunity and overall health.

Home Remedies Have Been Used for Years

The active ingredients in home remedies are organic. They are from organic plants, vegetables, fruits, and herbs. As such, they are easy to find, and using them is simple. You could use these home remedies, either raw or boiled. In some cases, they can also be boiled or even cooked.

Home Remedies Support a Healthy Lifestyle

When you choose to go for home remedies instead of prescription drugs, you promote a healthier lifestyle. Home remedies are especially helpful if you're a person who exercises regularly and is keen on watching your body fat as well as the amount of alcohol that goes into your body.

Home Remedies are Inexpensive

Pharmaceutical drugs are expensive, and the prices for these medications increase with each passing year. Whenever you buy them, the manufacturers get profits since you'll spend a lot. However, with home remedies, you get to save quite an amount.

Home Remedies are Milder

Since home remedies are fresher and more natural, they are pure in terms of medicinal content. As such, they directly attack your injury and cure it faster.

Home Remedies Have Fewer Side Effects

Pharmaceutical medications can have different side effects, such as drowsiness, skin irritation, among others. When you go for natural home remedies, the number of side effects you can experience is significantly reduced.

They Save You Frequent Visits to the Doctor

When you choose to go for natural home remedies, you will not need to go to the doctor for a prescription. Since they have few risks, figuring out how to go about using them is easier. They also provide a user-friendly option to prescription medicine from a doctor.

Disadvantages of Home Remedies

While there are so many advantages of using natural home remedies in healing injuries from home accidents, there are certain disadvantages of using them. They include:

It Takes Longer to See Results

While they are very effective, natural home remedies require you to have more patients compared to drugs you buy at a pharmacy. That's because their impact is not as immediate, and while you will heal, it will take a relatively long time compared to pharmaceutical drugs.

You Can't Be Sure of the Type of Treatment Needed

With home remedies, you do not really need to visit a doctor for an exam or prescription. As such, the treatment and its suitability are merely based on assumptions.

There's a Chance of the Wrong Dosage

With home remedies, you could either end up taking or using too much or too little. As such, an overdose, which is really dangerous, is highly possible.

Effectiveness of Some is not Proven

The advantage of pharmaceutical drugs is that they have undergone thorough testing. As such, their effectiveness in healing different injuries from home accidents is proven. However, the same cannot be said for natural home remedies. Not all of them have been proven to be effective.

Some Home Remedies Could be Poisonous

Since some of these natural home remedies are wild, they could lead to poisoning when taken orally or could cause poisoning to your skin or the eyes.

When it comes to domestic accidents, there are certain home remedies that you could use to ensure faster healing. Here are some of those home remedies:

Home Remedies for Cuts

Aloe Vera

Aloe vera has many benefits on one's body generally, but on cuts specifically, it has cooling properties and bears some substantial enzymes and vitamins that improve the health of your skin even after healing. Due to its anti-inflammatory properties, it helps reduce swelling quickly. The aloe vera leaves have a gel-like substance that contains several vitamins and minerals that help cuts heal much faster. The glucomannan present in aloe vera is effective in the regeneration of cells and the production of collagen, which speeds up the healing of wounds. Using it for cuts is very easy. All you have to do is apply a thin layer of the gel to the cut area or use a bandage that's been soaked in aloe vera gel to wrap the area.

Turmeric

It's very common to find turmeric in any kitchen. It's a humble spice that acts as a natural antiseptic and a natural antibiotic too. For many years, turmeric has been used for different medicinal purposes, and it works great on cuts. It has curcumin that's known to help in boosting wound healing. It does so through modulating the collagen. In case you're bleeding around the area of the cut, apply some turmeric, and you'll notice that the bleeding will stop almost immediately. To help the cut victim heal even faster, make them drink some turmeric milk every day before they sleep.

Honey

Another very effective home remedy for cuts is honey. Whenever you apply honey to a cut, it helps in dehydrating the bacteria present in it and helps in providing antibacterial help to the area. It's also known to boost tissue growth as it removes the dead tissues around the cut or wound area, facilitating faster healing. Honey has anti-bacterial, antimicrobial, antifungal, antiseptic, and anti-inflammatory properties, which is why it's been used for years in the treatment of wounds. Whenever you get a cut, just apply honey directly to it regularly. Its antioxidant and anti-bacterial property in honey keeps the wound moist. Since honey's viscosity is high, it goes a long way in providing a protective barrier on the wound and also prevents any microbial infections.

Garlic

Eating garlic is known to help in combating infections that can be caused by bacteria from the air or food. However, you could also apply it directly to cut wounds. Make a garlic paste and apply a layer of it to the area. This helps in treating any external infections. Garlic is known to have antimicrobial properties and anti-bacterial properties. As such, it helps in stopping the bleeding almost instantly. Garlic also helps reduce pain and promotes faster healing. All you have to do is apply a few garlic cloves, preferably crushed, on the cut or wound area.

Cinnamon

Cinnamon has anti-bacterial properties that are helpful in healing wounds from cuts. It is great for fighting infections and reducing inflammation. It's great to help out with healing much faster by cooling it.

Coconut Oil

Coconut oil has both anti-inflammatory and anti-bacterial properties. These help fight any infections that arise as a result of the cut, and just a simple application could help you heal faster and will keep your skin hydrated. Apply a few drops and then cover the wound with a piece of cloth two or three times a day for faster healing. Make sure the coconut oil you go for is of high quality.

Onions

Onions contain allicin, which is an antimicrobial compound known to prevent wounds from getting infected. They also have anti-inflammatory properties that are great for healing wounds. You could use a blend of both onions and honey as a paste on the cut. It will kill the bacteria before it ends up infecting your wound and help you heal even faster.

Limestone Powder

Limestone powder is sometimes known as chuna. It's also known to provide some healing properties and is easy to use on the cut wound area. Mix chuna and turmeric, heat them both, and apply the mixture on the wound for complete healing.

Cucumbers

Cucumbers are great in the healing of wounds because they're rich in vitamin A. The vitamin A activates collagen synthesis as it stimulates the inflammatory response of the body. This is helpful in the production of new tissue that replaces the damaged ones. It's also a source of silica that's known to help in the regrowth of connective body tissues. Cucumbers help in the maintaining of healthy blood pressure. As such, it facilitates the better flow of oxygen, vitamins, and the nutrients needed by the body, facilitating better wound healing.

Lavender

Essential oils such as lavender are known to work great on the skin. You can apply a drop or maybe two on the cut area so that it heals faster. Its anti-inflammatory properties are great in the reduction of swelling and the healing of cuts. It also has antimicrobial properties that prevent the occurrence of any bacterial infections.

Peppermint Oil

Peppermint oil is great in the relief of pain. Simply apply the oil on the affected area but ensure you keep it off the broken skin. Do not apply it directly to the wound.

Tea Tree Oil

Tea tree oil, as well as being great for healing skin conditions, is also great in healing open wounds and different types of cuts. It has a lot of anti-inflammatory properties, and applying a drop of it will help you heal faster from it.

Cayenne Pepper

Cayenne pepper has been used for years in Asia as medicine. You need to crush it into a powder then apply it directly on the cut. It's antibacterial and antifungal properties will give relief to the affected area. When you're bleeding, you can mix the cayenne powder with some water, as this will equalize the blood pressure. After that, you will be able to slow down the flow of blood and allow it to clot.

Chamomile Tea

Chamomile tea also has the anti-inflammatory properties or antimicrobial ones required in the healing of cuts.

Cloves

Cloves, aside from having anti-inflammatory properties, also have analgesic components. Cloves are, therefore, effective in battling infection around the cut area and in stopping the infection from spreading.

Apple Cider Vinegar

Apple cider vinegar is very helpful in preventing the growth of bacteria in the area where the cut is. Its acidic nature creates a great environment for killing bacteria. However, you should dilute it with water before using it.

Home Remedies for Burns

Burns can be very painful, so people usually search for things that may soothe the pain as a home remedy. However, keeping the burned tissue properly hydrated and protected from infections is the top priority, so it's important to avoid any "home remedies" that are popular among people and, however, ineffective and rather dangerous to the burned person.

Home Remedies to Avoid

These are the home remedies you shouldn't use, no matter what anyone tells you about treating burns at home:

- Mint Toothpaste

- Coconut Oil

- Vinegar

- Vanilla

- Teabags

- Milk

- Oats

- Lavender Oil

- Onions or any other vegetables

Home Remedies to Use

These are the home remedies that are not only safe to use in burns, but also beneficial.

- Aloe Vera Gel: It prevents inflammation, reduces the pain, stimulates skin growth and repair, and it's safe.

- Honey: It's only safe to use medical-grade honey because it's sterile, and you can only use it in minor first-degree burns. It soothes pain and reduces inflammation.

- Antibiotic Creams: These are the standard treatment for burn injuries. Silver sulfadiazine cream is particularly effective and recommended for such injuries. Once the burnt area has been hydrated, it should be covered with an antibiotic cream to reduce the risk of infection.

- Vitamin C and Vitamin E: Vitamin C is mostly associated with colds. However, it has many more benefits than just that. Vitamin C helps in the healing of wounds much faster and in producing more collagen. Collagen acts as a base material for the development of new skin. To help your burn heal faster, eat food that is rich in vitamin C and also vitamin E. You can also take about two thousand milligrams of vitamin C and about 1000 IU of vitamin E for seven days after your burn accident. Another thing you can do is break the vitamin E capsule and directly apply it to the burn. This will help in healing, and even better, it will ensure there is no scarring.

- •Over-the-Counter Pain Medication: Burns are very painful, and that's why a burn victim might prefer to take some medication for the burn until they heal. This medication could also help reduce swelling, aside from just the pain. Over-the-counter medication like ibuprofen is both safe and effective in achieving this as it's a non-steroidal drug that will decrease inflammation.

Home Remedies for Bruises

Whenever you have a bruise, you could use the following remedies:

Ice Therapy

When an injury gives you a bruise, get some ice, and immediately apply it to the bruised area. It will help reduce the blood flow there and cool the blood vessels. Cooling the vessels is important in reducing the amount of blood leaking into the surrounding tissue. As a result, the bruise will be less apparent, and any swelling in the area will significantly go down. For this, you could go for a reusable ice pack, a bag of frozen vegetables, or some ice in a bag. For all of these, wrap them in a towel before placing them on the skin. Ice the bruised area for ten minutes at a time. Remember to give it some time, preferably twenty minutes before you apply the pack again.

Use Heat

You can also apply some heat to the bruised area to heal it. Heat boosts circulation on the bruised area and also increases the flow of blood in it. When you do this, the trapped blood, which is a result of the bruise, will clear away. Heat is also useful in loosening any tense muscles and in relieving pain. For this, a heating pad or a bottle of hot water will be useful. You can also soak in a hot bath for the same effect.

Compression

You should wrap the bruised area properly in an elastic bandage. It will help squeeze the tissues and will prevent leaking of the blood vessels. Compression is very useful in lessening the bruise's severity and in the reduction of pain and swelling in the area.

Elevation

You could also keep the bruised area elevated above the heart. This will help relieve pain and in draining the fluid left in the bruised area. When you elevate the bruised area, you also help reduce pressure, and this will allow you or the victim to rest and relax. This, in turn, facilitates faster healing.

Arnica

Arnica is a homeopathic kind of herb that's useful in reducing inflammation and any kind of swelling that is caused by bruises. Whenever you apply it on any bruises induced by lasers a number of times within the day, you'll find that healing will take place within a shorter period. There's also the option of orally taking arnica to heal bruises faster.

Vitamin K Cream

Vitamin K is useful in blood clotting, and because of this, it goes a long way in making bruises less severe. To use it effectively, apply the vitamin K gently, rubbing it on the bruises at least twice a day.

Vitamin C

When you eat foods that are rich in vitamin C, or when you take supplements rich in vitamin C, you'll heal faster from bruises. Vitamin C helps fight inflammation. You can also apply creams rich in vitamin C directly in the bruise.

Quercetin

Quercetin is a flavonoid with natural anti-inflammatory properties that are obtained from different fruits. It can heal bruises faster. You can usually find some creams or gels that contain quercetin, which you could just apply based on the directions on the packaging. Doing so twice daily will significantly improve the appearance of the bruised area and will promote faster healing. You should avoid orally taking quercetin as there are some issues regarding its safety. It can also get mixed up with other medications, which could be harmful. Before you take any quercetin supplements, seek medical advice from a health professional.

Bromelain

Bromelain is made up of a mixture of certain enzymes present in the pineapple plant. These enzymes contain anti-inflammatory properties that significantly help in reducing bruises and any swelling when it's applied to the bruised area. For better results, it's advisable to apply bromelain about two to three times a day unless you've been directed otherwise. You should only take bromelain orally when directed by a doctor. People who get allergic reactions after eating pineapples should avoid bromelain.

Comfrey

Comfrey is a plant that comes in handy when it comes to healing different kinds of skin issues and inflammation. It's been proven to treat bruises. Apply the comfrey cream a few times a day on the bruise. Another option is to create a compress. For this, use dry comfrey leaves. Steep them in boiling water for about ten minutes then strain the liquid out. Wrap the leaves inside a towel or a clean piece of cloth then apply it to the bruise.

Eating a Proper Diet

What you eat can go a long way in improving the appearance of your bruise and even in healing it all together. Some foods are known to strengthen the blood vessels, which subsequently reduces bruising while others are great for the skin. They improve the skin and other tissues. You should, therefore, eat foods that are nutritious and always aim for a balanced diet. The following foods can help in either the prevention or healing of bruises:

- Foods that naturally contain quercetin. These foods include red onion, berries, especially the dark-colored ones, apples, cherries, and green leafy vegetables.

- Citrus fruits such as tangerines, oranges, and lemons. These help in healing bruises, especially among the elderly.

- Pineapples. Eating pineapples means you naturally get bromelain that facilitates faster healing of bruises.

- Vitamin K –rich foods. When you eat a diet that's rich in vitamin K, you will make your body stronger and less likely to get bruised. Some foods that are packed with vitamin K include kales, broccoli, spinach, soybeans, lettuce, blueberries, and strawberries.

- Foods rich in zinc such as crabs, lobster, pumpkin seeds, legumes, and spinach. These greatly help in healing the tissues and wounds.

- Lean protein. Protein-rich foods such as tofu, lean meat, and fish greatly help in strengthening capillaries. Stay away from protein foods that contain saturated fats in high amounts.

Essential Oils

Essential oils, such as frankincense, can relieve pain and help you relax. For best results, mix it with some vitamin K and arnica. Similarly, you could ease the pain of a bruise by creating a cold compress that will soothe the injuries using a few drops of lavender and rosemary essential oils applied on a washcloth then to the bruised area. It's advisable that instead of using the essential oils directly on your skin, you dilute them with carrier lotion to avoid skin irritation unless you have been directed otherwise by a health professional.

Home Remedies for Sprains

Getting a sprain can slow you down and ruin your routine. However, some home remedies could help you heal faster from it.

Ice

When you first suffer a sprain, the first great thing you can do to help yourself is cryotherapy. A cold compress on the sprain injury is known to speed up the process of healing. You should, however, be careful not to overdo it; otherwise, you risk getting frostbite. Use gel packs to do ice compresses routinely and make sure the ice stays on for just as long as is required, twenty minutes at a time. Should you feel that the ice is getting too cold for you to bear before the twenty minutes are up, just keep the ice on the sprain for a period that's alright for you.

Compression

If you want your sprain to heal even faster, compression will help. A brace or a wrap will, to a great extent, stop further swelling and will also give you that much-needed stability as it puts pressure on the injured part.

Elevation

Elevation is also another simple way through which you can make the healing process of your sprain faster. Every time you sit down, or when you're lying and have a sprained ankle, prop it up so that it rests above your heart or your waist to reduce swelling. Elevating your ankle prevents the buildup of unwanted fluids around the sprained area. Whenever you start to feel a little restless, grab the opportunity to relax and prop your ankles up.

Rest and Exercising

Whenever you get a sprain, you need to make sure you get enough rest; otherwise, you risk making the situation even worse. Once you have recovered or if you feel better, do not be too quick to go back to your normal activities. Instead, seek medical advice first as you might need some physical therapy. You will need to find a balance between exercising and resting so that you do not overwork the injured area. Pushing too hard could end up weakening the area.

Onions

Whenever you have a sprain, grate an onion, add some salt to it, then gently place on the sprained part. Use gauze to wrap around it so that the mixture remains in place. You can, therefore, use some plastic around it to ensure the mixture remains moist. You should then take a bandage and use it to hold everything in place for about eight hours. In some cases, you will need to repeat the exact same procedure. The onions will allow your blood vessels to open up, which will reduce swelling, bruising, and congestion properly.

Epsom Salt

After a few days of spraining your ankle, for example, you can soak the sprained area in a warm bath that contains some Epsom salt. Epsom salt is known to be effective in soothing sore muscles in the body and connective tissues too. It helps in easing the stiffness, and you should, therefore, use it about twice a day.

Over-the-Counter Medication

A sprain might not be the typical kind of injury, but it does bring some pain. In case this pain is too much to handle, go for some over-the-counter pain medication. This will help in reducing the swelling and the pain. However, if you're already taking some kind of medication, seek a doctor's advice first.

Garlic

Garlic is also helpful in healing ankle sprains. It calms the pain significantly and improves the injury's recovery time. Garlic also generally strengthens your immune system. Using it is very easy.

Clean the sprained area then dry it properly. Make some garlic juice and take a tablespoon of it. Mix with some almond or coconut oil then gently massage it on the injured area for about ten minutes. Clean the area well after this and make sure you repeat this process twice daily for about two to three weeks.

Olive Oil

Olive oil has some phenomenal materials that help alleviate inflammation. It's also helpful in quickening the healing process. Use a teaspoon to take some olive oil and then heat it. Leave it for a few minutes to cool, but not completely. You need it warm. Massage it gently onto the sprained area for a while. For best results, do this three times a day. It will help your muscles relax. Another way you can go about it is by mixing some of the olive oil with egg yolk then smearing the mixture on the sprained area. Use a clean piece of cloth to wrap the area for two days. After that, remove the piece of cloth and repeat the process in case you still don't feel better.

Turmeric

Turmeric is not only a great spice, but it's also a home remedy that can help in the alleviation of different kinds of pains and inflammation from sprains. Turmeric prevents blood from clotting and improves the flow of blood. You just need to mix the turmeric powder with some warm water until the consistency resembles that of a balm. Into this mixture, add some lemon juice and hit the mixture. Smear it on the area that has been sprained and then wrap it. Take the wrap or bandage off. You should repeat this process for three continuous days. Turmeric can also be taken orally. Mix some milk with some turmeric powder and then drink it two times a day.

Castor Oil

Castor oil contains some amino acids that are packed with anti-inflammatory properties. The extraordinary amino acid in castor oil is called oxalic acid and has been used for years in treating ankle issues. To use it, grab a bowl and in it pour some castor oil then dip a piece of cotton cloth inside. Use the piece of cloth on the hurt area and add a bandage around it. Heat some water and then transfer it into a rubber water bottle. Place the hot water bottle on the sprained area and leave it there for thirty minutes. Make sure you keep your leg lifted. Remove the bottle and the bandage and then give the area a good massage. For best results, do this three times a day for about two to three days.

Ginger Roots

The roots of ginger plants are great for reducing the symptoms of sprains, such as swelling and pain. To use it, take a pot and fill it with eight cups of water. Cut a ginger root of between two to three inches long and add to the water. For five minutes, boil the water then turn off the source of heat. Let the water sit until it cools to room temperature. Take a clean piece of cotton cloth and dip it in the ginger water, then use it to wrap the sprained area. For best results, make sure you start treating the sprain using this method within two or three days of the time you got the sprain. You should also avoid using the water when it's too hot, as it might end up irritating your skin.

Cabbage

Cabbage also has anti-inflammatory properties that can help in then reducing of pain around the sprained area. It contains phytonutrients and vitamins, which are compounds that help in the faster healing of the injury. You only need to remove the cabbage's outer leaves then squeeze the juice from them. Heat the squeezed leaves in the oven for a few minutes while they're covered in tin foil. Place them on the sprained area and then use a bandage to cover both the leaves and the area. To ensure that the area remains properly warmed, cover the sprained area using a blanket for about thirty minutes. Do this two times a day for two days.

Magnesium Sulfate

Magnesium sulfate is a kind of mineral salt that is readily available in pharmacies. It's also called English salt and can be used externally to treat different kinds of skin ailments and inflammations. It's also helpful in treating sprained ankles. Take a cup and fill it with some magnesium salt then pour the salt in a tub containing some lukewarm water. Mix the water properly so that the magnesium salt crystals melt in it completely. You should then soak the sprained area for half an hour and repeat the process twice a day for about three days.

Chapter 17

Over-the-Counter Medication in Treating Domestic Accidents

Sometimes, when people become victims of domestic accidents, they go for over-the-counter medication to heal them.

Benefits of Over-the-Counter Medication

Here are some benefits of over-the-counter medication for home injuries:

They are Convenient

Over-the-counter medication does not require one to go for a consultation to a doctor before use. All you have to do is research on the common ones for things such as pain or swelling, among others. After this, you could go to a local pharmacy and just purchase it. If you're not sure about the medication you need for a given domestic accident, you could always ask the pharmacist, and they'll be able to advise you on the best one to go for.

They are Readily Available

It's so easy to get over-the-counter medication. They are not only sold in pharmacies but also in shops, supermarkets, and other places. That's why many people prefer them whenever domestic accidents happen, and they would like to help the victim in case they are in any pain.

They are Easy to Understand

Over-the-counter medications usually have very few instructions to follow, which make them user-friendly, especially when the domestic accident victim is in pain and needs some urgent help.

They are Inexpensive

Over-the-counter drugs are usually less costly compared to prescription drugs. The process of acquiring them is also inexpensive as you do not have to pay consultation fees at the doctor's like you would have paid to get prescription drugs.

They Give People a Sense of Control Over Their Lives

With over-the-counter medication, you get to decide what to take for your condition. You can, for example, pick the type of painkiller based on how much money you have and the amount of pain as well as the strength of the individual painkiller brands. They are mostly taken depending on the victim's current state.

Disadvantages of Over-the-Counter Drugs

While over-the-counter drugs help in treating and healing injuries from domestic accidents, they also have certain disadvantages which include:

There's a Risk of Taking the Wrong Medication

Most of the time, over-the-counter drugs are taken based on the assumption of what the extent of the injury is. They don't involve lab tests, doctor's consultations, or x-rays. As such, one risks taking the wrong medication.

There's a Risk of an Overdose

Just as there is the risk of taking the wrong medication, you could actually overdose on the drugs, especially when you take them more times than you should in a day or if you take the medication at the wrong intervals. Sometimes, some people end up taking more than they should, which can pose a bigger health threat.

You Could Develop an Allergic Reaction or Experience Poisoning

Most people are not too keen on checking the ingredients that make up certain over-the-counter medication. As such, they end up taking medication to heal injuries that are a result of domestic accidents, but the medication brings about another problem. It could trigger allergic reactions or, even worse, lead to poisoning when taken in the wrong quantity. People with certain underlying health conditions should also avoid certain drugs. The risk of overdose is also present because some companies that manufacture those over-the-counter drugs use multiple ingredients to make the medication usable for different kinds of symptoms. The problem with this is that most consumers do not need to have all those active ingredients in their bodies, so this just increases their risk of getting intoxicated.

Taking Them Could Cause Discomfort or Long-Term Illnesses

You could develop some feelings of discomfort when you take certain over-the-counter drugs. For example, you might end up with an upset stomach, diarrhea, among others. Certain over-the-counter drugs, when taken for a long time, could end up causing long-term medical conditions such as kidney failure, liver damage, or heart problems.

Factors to Consider When Buying or Taking Over-the-Counter Drugs

Having discussed the benefits and dangers of using over-the-counter drugs in the treatment or healing process after being a domestic accident victim, here are some factors to consider before buying or taking them:

Label and Ingredients

Some medications are very common, and because of this, a lot of people often take them simply for their popularity. However, just because you've seen a drug being used often does not mean it's right for you. Make it a point to always check the labels on the packaging of the medication. Read them carefully to avoid consuming drugs that have serious side effects. Make sure you don't ignore any of the warnings that are written on those labels. They'll help you know when to use the drug when to take a break or stop using it completely.

They'll also give you information on whether or not to see a doctor should any side effects arise.

Check the active ingredients that are on the label, the purpose of the product, and the product category. Is it an antihistamine, cough suppressant, antacid? Check the uses of the medication, the other symptoms or diseases this product will treat. Check the storage information so that you know how to ensure it's always safe to take. It's also always worth checking the active ingredients in the drug, such as the colors and the flavoring.

Even if you trust in the strength of your eyesight, always ensure that you're in a well-lit room whenever you're reading the labels.

Also, read the product name well. Just because you find two over-the-counter drugs with an almost similar name does not mean they treat the same condition. Also, just because you find different kinds of medication with a similar brand name does not mean they're supposed to treat the same medical condition.

In case you have read the label but are still uncertain about something, make sure you ask a pharmacist or a doctor.

Its Interaction with Your Body

Sometimes, medication interacts with our bodies in a way that's not normal. As such, it's very important to observe carefully how your body interacts with a given drug. Here are some precautions to take in order to avoid certain drug interactions:

Stay away from alcohol whenever you are under any kind of medication, especially if they contain ingredients such as dextromethorphan. Even if you're in pain from a domestic accident, stay away from drugs that treat sleeplessness if you're already taking any prescription sedatives. You should also check with a doctor if it's safe to take any over-the-counter drugs that contain aspirin if you're already taking prescribed blood thinners or if you have a condition such as gout. Avoid laxatives if you're experiencing some kind of nausea from a domestic accident.

Underlying Medical Conditions

You should consider any medical conditions like high blood pressure, diabetes, and the likes before you take any over-the-counter medication because the over-the-counter medication could, instead of treating your pain, cause more harm. If you suffer from any condition, always consult a doctor before taking certain over-the-counter drugs. This is to ensure that the drugs you're taking do not collide with the ones you're taking.

The Dosage

It's always important to follow any instructions given with regards to dosage, especially if the domestic accident victim you're administering the medication to is a child. They are more vulnerable. Measurements are very important and should not be underestimated. Therefore, do not add or reduce the amount even if you're giving it to a child. You should also make sure you do not administer or take two medications that are supposed to cure one illness.

The Seal

You should always check to see if the seal of your medication is in good condition or if it's been tampered with. If you find that the seal is broken, it could mean that the drug was tampered with. You should, therefore, always inspect the packaging of the medication and what's inside to see if everything's fine.

Other precautions to take with over-the-counter drugs include checking your over-the-counter medication cabinet. Many people have these just in case an accident happens at home. You should:

- Check your medication supply at least once a year to ensure you throw out any that might be expired and replace any that you might have run out of

- Check that your storage area for them is cool and dry unless otherwise stated on the labels of the medication

- Keep all the medication labeled and in their original containers so that no one ends up taking the wrong ones

In case a pregnant or a breastfeeding mother is the victim of a domestic accident, take extra precaution in case you're thinking of using over-the-counter medication. That's because a dosage might be alright for the mother, but at the same time, it could be harmful to the unborn baby. So, if you're pregnant, always call your doctor and ask them first before you take any over-the-counter drugs.

In case you're breastfeeding, remember that it's easy for drugs to pass into your breast milk. Luckily, the concentration of these drugs is usually low in these cases and might not necessarily harm your baby. However, it's always worth calling your doctor or a pharmacist and asking them about it before you proceed to take these drugs. They will give you information on the best times to take these drugs and could also give you valuable directions on how to adjust the dosage so that both you and the child remain safe.

When it Comes to Children, Remember

- Not to base the dosage on their size. Medications are not created based on the children's sizes, so stick to the instructions given to the latter. The goal is to help them heal from domestic accidents and not to make the situation worse

- It's important to read the label carefully and follow all the directions especially if there are any on age limits

- Some OTC drugs come in different strengths so what might be safe for an older child could be unsafe for a younger one and what could be suitable for a younger child might not have an effect on an older child

- Remember that there's a big difference between TBSP (tablespoon) and TSP (teaspoon). Both of them give very different doses. If the label says, for example, give two teaspoons, it's better to measure using just that. A teaspoon so that you avoid estimating the amount you're administering

- Never play doctor. Just because a child seems sicker does not mean you're free to double the dose of medication they're taking.

- Before you decide to give your child two different medications at the same time, ensure you talk to the pharmacist. Give them all the information regarding your child's domestic accident and ask any questions you may have

- Do not allow your child to take medication by themselves and never call any medication candy because should they come across it while you're not around, they might end up taking it

Another great precaution to take is to go for child-resistant packaging. Child-resistant closures are great for your home's OTC counter as they ensure you have medication on standby while they also make it difficult for your child to open them in case they're unattended for a while. In any case, always make sure you store all medication far away from children's reach. Never leave medication containers on counters where they'll be visible. You should also avoid hiding medication in briefcases and purses. Remember, children are also good at copying what they see adults doing, so if you're taking any medication after a domestic accident, don't do it in front of children. They might be tempted to do exactly what you did when you least expect it.

You should also protect yourself from tampering when you're getting any over-the-counter drug for domestic accidents by checking to see if there are any tamper-evident features, inspecting the packaging then inspecting the medication too when you get home. In case the medication looks discolored, do not use it. If you notice anything suspicious, avoid taking the medication too.

Chapter 18

Seeking Professional Treatment

D omestic accidents can be very serious, and in some cases, first aid and home remedies are not enough to help the situation. As such, you may need to call or get to a medical professional for help, better diagnosis, and faster healing. This could involve calling an ambulance or going straight to the doctor's office by yourself if you're the victim or if you're the one taking care of the accident victim.

Why You Should Call an Ambulance After a Domestic Accident

Some domestic accidents are usually more serious than others, and as such, it is highly recommended that you call an ambulance for medical transportation. Some of the reasons why you should call an ambulance include:

It's a Life-Saving Alternative

In the event that the domestic accident victim's life is on the line, calling an ambulance could save their life as the trained personnel will get to your exact location and offer initial assistance. Throughout the trip to the hospital, the victim will still be under observation. Remember, time is very crucial when there's a victim badly hurt, and if you're driving the victim yourself, the outcome could be deadly. An ambulance, on the other hand, is allowed to travel faster on the roads ensuring the victim gets to the hospital in good time for treatment. Another great thing about an ambulance is that it can alert the emergency department to be ready to receive the accident victim.

Ambulances are Safe and Convenient

Since an ambulance is meant specifically for medical transportation, it ensures the victim of a domestic accident is safe.

Signs That You Should Call an Ambulance

Certain situations require you to call an ambulance. They include:

- If the victim of the domestic accident already has a life-threatening condition

- If there's a chance that the condition of the victim could get worse when you're at home or on the way to the hospital

- In cases where moving the domestic accident victim could cause further injury to them

- If traffic could prevent you from getting to the hospital in good time

Things to observe when calling an ambulance

When you decide to call an ambulance, it's important to observe the following:

- Remain calm and speak slowly so that you are able to relay the message about the domestic accident clearly

- Listen carefully to all the questions the dispatcher is asking you

- Always give your full name so that it is well recorded

- Give the exact address of the place where the accident victim is

- Always give the phone number you're using, especially if you're using a cell phone for the call. It makes it easier for the ambulance service to reach you in case any further information is needed when the ambulance is on the way

- Give further details on the location of the victim, for example, are they upstairs, in the garden, back yard, bathroom, etc.

- Explain the exact nature of the problem. What happened to the victim? Are they responsive? Are they breathing properly?

- Make sure you stay on the line until the dispatcher tells you it's alright to hang up. Hanging up too soon is not advised as the dispatcher might need additional information or to give you instructions to follow as you wait

The following are ways to tell between a real emergency and a minor issue. Real emergencies involve:

- Difficulty in breathing or if the victim has shortness of breath. Check to see if the victim looks like they're sucking in below their rib cage or if they are using other body muscles to help them breathe

- Chest pain, pressure or pain in the upper abdomen of the victim's body

- Fainting of the victim

- Feelings of sudden dizziness or if the victim feels very weak. If their vision changes too, there could be something more serious happening to their body

- A change in their normal mental state for example, if they feel confused or if they're behaving unusually

- Suddenly feeling severe pain in any part of the body after the accident

- The victim bleeding profusely and you can't stop it even by applying direct pressure to the injury

- Persistent vomiting by the victim, coughing or if they start vomiting blood

- The patient is suicidal all of a sudden or has homicidal feelings

- The victim is experiencing seizures for the first time and the fits last for more than three minutes

- The victim is experiencing severe allergic reactions that are unusual

Here are some more things to do to be prepared for an emergency situation

- Post different emergency phone numbers of the police, fire department, poison control, and physicians near the phones in your house or compound. You should also print out a list of the same.

- You can post a list of directions alongside them too. These directions will be helpful in case you start to panic when an accident actually happens, as you could just look at them and follow the instructions. These directions are also helpful in case there is a child at home who can read. They could always follow the instructions in the absence of an adult

- Teach young children how to call for help in case of different domestic accidents, whether using a landline or a cell phone

- Ensure that your house number is clear and well posted to make it easier for the ambulance to find you when they get to the area the accident occurred

- It's also worth leaving the porch light on even if it's not night time as it makes it easier for the ambulance to find your correct location. If there's someone else with you, have them meet the ambulance

- If the victim has been taking any medication, ensure you gather all of them in one place and give them to the ambulance team for inspection. In case you're unable to gather all of them, write a list of all the medication the victim takes

- Leave the victim as they are, meaning you should not help them shower or dress them as you wait to have them transferred to the hospital. You should also avoid dressing them as the ambulance crew will have to access their chest, arms, and abdomen to check for blood pressure and to conduct an electrocardiogram

- In case you have a pet, whether friendly or not, put it in a different room. Pets are known to turn hostile whenever they see strangers bursting into the room. They could subsequently get in the way of the ambulance crew setting up their equipment and providing the medical care needed to bring the victim to safety

- If you can, have someone help you move all the furniture away. Make sure the stairway and the floors are clear so that the ambulance crew can bring in the stretcher and the rest of their equipment without struggling

- Make sure the area where the victim is has good lighting. Turn the lights on in that room and on the path that will be used by the ambulance crew

- The accident crew will most likely need to use oxygen to help the victim breathe. As such, you should ensure cigarettes are turned off and do the same to all other smoking items

- Ensure there is a wastebasket at the scene of the accident just in case certain things need to be thrown away to clear the area

- Always keep a key hidden outside your house. In case you're the accident victim, and the door is locked, you can always tell the ambulance crew where the key is located if you can't get up and open the door by yourself.

Things to Remember When You Choose To Use an Ambulance

People often expect certain things when they use ambulance services. However, these may not be a true reflection of the way things work.

- When you get to the hospital, you will not automatically be the first to get medical attention in the emergency room. It is definitely not interesting to wait in the triage area. However, the staff at the hospital will usually prioritize by the need of the patients and not the mode of transport they used to get to the hospital.

- You might have a preference for a given hospital. However, the ambulance might not take you there. They will always try to be as accommodating as possible; however, they have to consider several factors before deciding on which hospital to take the patient to. For example, your preferred hospital might be too crowded to accommodate the accident victim that they are directed to go elsewhere. In other cases, they might have to take the victim to the nearest hospital because of bad weather or the high number of calls coming in of people requesting their services.

- Remember that as much as the ambulance crew is well trained to handle medical emergencies, they are neither hospitals on wheels nor doctors. Do not expect them to make a full diagnosis of the situation. They cannot perform x-rays on the injured areas or tell you when the victim will fully recover. All they do is give emergency care. So you have to wait until you get to a hospital to get your questions answered.

- While ambulances are expected to arrive at an emergency scene quickly, certain factors like your geographical location could cause a delay in the response time. This is especially true if you live in a rural area. In case you live in a city, heavy traffic could cause a delay too.

Reasons to See a Doctor After a Domestic Injury

You or a victim of a domestic accident might feel fine after some first aid treatment, but in some cases, it's still important to see a doctor. Here are some reasons why:

To Find Out the Extent of the Injury

A domestic accident such as a fall, getting hit by a falling object, and the likes could seem like something one would easily recover from, but in some cases, the injury could be more serious than what meets the eye. So even if the accident victim feels alright at the moment, it's worth going to see a doctor for further examinations just to confirm that there really isn't too much to worry about. In case there is a serious injury, it will be detected sooner and treated so that it does not bring any more issues in the future. Internal injuries are not usually visible and, as such, are hard to detect, but if soft tissue injuries are left untreated for long, they could lead to severe pain.

To Get Effective Treatment at a Lower Cost

Many people assume that they're just sore and will easily ignore the pain from a domestic accident. However, there is a risk in doing this because in case the injury is worse than you think, then you're not getting the right treatment. As such, the problem could worsen and could end up impacting your way of life negatively. You will then end up paying higher medical bills than you would have if you had just received effective treatment from the start.

To Get the Right Prescription Drugs

We've talked about over-the-counter medication, and while it has several benefits, it's better to see a doctor because they give you medication to take according to the actual results of the examination and not based on assumptions. You will also be able to get the medication in the right dosage.

Signs the Accident Victim Needs a Doctor

There are certain signs to generally look out for after an accident. When you see them, you need to take the victim to the hospital.

A Persistent Fever

Generally, a fever shows the natural way in which your body fights the different types of infections. However, when it's too high, it's cause for alarm. If, after the accident, fever lasts more than three days, the accident victim needs to see a doctor.

Shortness of Breath

Sometimes, depending on the type of accident, the victim could have shortness of breath which, if not professionally addressed immediately, could lead to further complications, and the victim could end up critical. In some cases, it can be fatal. Breathing problems should never be ignored.

Bright Flashes and Interruption in Vision

If, after the accident, the victim experiences strong migraines, bright flashes, and spots in their vision, it could be a sign of a more serious injury. They might need to see a doctor sooner rather than later.

When the Victim's Mood Changes Suddenly or They Experience Confusion

When an accident victim suddenly experiences confusion or sudden changes in their mood, you should take them to see a doctor. Symptoms of some injuries, such as head injuries sometimes don't appear until many hours after the actual accident.

When You Suspect a Concussion

In case you've fallen at home, especially on your head, and suffered a blow to it, you need to monitor your progress of healing and be alert for symptoms of a concussion. The symptoms include severe headache, a change in the patterns of your sleep, irritability, among others. You should see a doctor immediately if you experience such problems.

In the Case of Chest Pains, Abdominal or Pelvic Ones

When after an accident, the victim experiences abnormal and intense pain that does not seem to go away in the chest area or the pelvis, it could be a sign of an underlying issue that needs the attention of a doctor as soon as possible.

Certain tests can be conducted by doctors whenever people have been hurt. They include:

X-rays

An x-ray is an electromagnetic radiation type or can be a type of electromagnetic wave. It's a way of taking pictures of the different bones in a patient's body to find fractures. The radiation penetrates through the soft tissues like fat, the skin, and muscles and makes broken bones easy to see.

CT Scan

A CT scan is short for a computed tomography scan. It's a type of x-ray, except it creates images of bones, soft tissue, internal organs, and blood vessels. It creates images that are more detailed and can be viewed in many different plans. As such, they generate images in three dimensions. While x-rays use a straight beam of radiation targeted to one body part, CT scans use multiple beams from different directions aimed at just one body part. Sometimes, the doctor will use a CT scan containing contrast. Contrast is when the patient is injected with dye or drinks contrast so that certain body parts are more visible in the images obtained. The CT scan machine is a circle that's doughnut-shaped, whereby a patient is slid into the "hole" of the donut. So, for the accident victim, the CT scan is used to show internal bleeding, broken bones, or injuries to the internal organs.

MRI

An MRI is a third kind of test that's usually ordered by doctors whenever someone's been hurt in an accident. It stands for Magnetic Resonance Imaging. It works through a magnetic field and radio waves pulses through the body and produces pictures. For these images to be produced, the patients are placed in enclosed tubes for several minutes, usually up to twenty or more. Just like a CT scan, the patients are often injected with dye to make a certain body part more visible. MRIs are useful in the diagnosis of neck and back injuries, bulging, or herniated discs, etc.

Prescription Medication in Healing Domestic Accidents

When you consult a doctor after a domestic accident, they will examine you, make a diagnosis then prescribe some medication.

Types of Prescription Drugs

Opioids

These are drugs that naturally occur in the poppy plant that produces opium. These kinds of prescription drugs are commonly referred to as painkillers. When you've been a victim of a domestic accident, a doctor will prescribe these as they block the pain signals between your body and the brain. Doctors prescribe opioids as a way of treating both moderate and severe pain levels.

Benzodiazepines

These are psychoactive drugs prescribed by doctors to domestic accident victims as a way of inhibiting or depressing certain processes of the central nervous system. They help a victim recover from any anxiety or panic attacks they may have as a result of the accident. However, they can also treat conditions like nausea, insomnia, seizures, and muscle relaxation.

Non-Benzodiazepine Sedatives

In case you end up suffering from insomnia as a result of the domestic accident, a doctor will prescribe these. They work by raising the level of amino acid Gamma-Aminobutyric Acid, which subsequently slows down the activity in the brain. This allows your mind and body to relax and helps promote sleep, which is needed for the body to heal.

Benefits of Prescription Drugs

When a doctor prescribes the medication for you, some of the benefits include:

You Get the Right Medication

Often, a doctor will examine you thoroughly to find out the extent of the injury. This ensures that they prescribe suitable medication for your exact condition so that you heal faster from it. They'll make sure the medication you take is just right in case you have any other underlying conditions or if you fall within a certain age bracket.

The Medication is Given in the Right Dosage

With prescription medication, the dosage is carefully indicated. The doctors and pharmacists are keen on explaining why you need to take that medication at a specific time and in a specific amount to facilitate healing. They will also tell you the period of time within which you should take the drugs and when to discontinue them and how quickly you should see results.

The Medications Will Rarely React with Each Other

Since doctors are trained in medicine, they are able to predict reactions prescription medication can have. For example, if you are already taking certain prescription medications for a given condition, they will anticipate the reactions that can arise from giving you certain painkillers. They, therefore, make sure you're safe from them. They will also be keen not to prescribe two different medications that do not mix well together.

Healing is Faster

With prescription medication, you can heal faster from the accident compared to home remedies and even over-the-counter medication.

Disadvantages of Getting Prescription Medication

They can be Costly

Compared to home remedies, the prescription medication cost is on the higher side owing to the ingredients they contain and the process involved in manufacturing them. In some cases, this could be the reason why some domestic accident victims get OTC medication instead.

They Require Consultation with a Doctor

For prescription drugs, you have to schedule an appointment with a doctor, visit an walk in clinic or emergency center.

The Prescription Medication Can Have Side Effects

When you take certain prescription drugs, they can cause side effects like drowsiness or hallucinations or even more serious side effects if you fail to take them per the doctor's instructions. That's because these prescription drugs are very specific in what they treat and in how they work, so you need to be really careful about how you use them.

How to Stay Safe When Using Prescription Medication for Domestic Accidents

While prescription medication is great, seeing that a doctor usually gives it, there are certain things you could do to ensure that you stay safe when using them to treat domestic accidents. They include:

- Keeping a comprehensive list of all the medications you take, whether prescription, herbal or over-the-counter. Also, have a list of all the types of medications you're allergic to, and beside the name, write down your allergy symptoms. This ensures that if you're brought to the hospital, for example, after an accident, and you can't speak, the doctors can assist you accordingly.

- Always ensure you take your medication only as recommended by a doctor. Read and follow all the instructions on the label or the instruction booklet of the medication. Make sure you have listened to the instructions given by the doctor and pharmacist in addition to the ones already indicated.

- In case you do not understand something about the prescription drug, ensure you ask your doctor or the pharmacist.

- Always take the medication in the correct amount. Avoid taking more than the recommended amount even if you're in a lot of pain.

- Avoid taking medication in the dark. Ensure you're doing so in a well-lit room so that you read the label correctly, and you measure the medication accurately.

- Never use a prescription medication that's prescribed for someone else, even if you feel like you have the same symptoms. No two cases or bodies are exactly the same.

- If you get prescription medication, always be aware of the fact that it can react with other medications. You should also be aware that different medications can end up reacting differently with certain fruits or food as well as alcoholic beverages. So, make sure you discuss the kind of medication you're taking in-depth with the physician so that you determine beforehand if any potential problems exist with the medication you're taking. Always check the labels.

- Never take old medications even if you feel like you're suffering or experiencing the same kind of pain from your accident as you previously did before.

- When you get new medication for your accident, ensure that you dispose of any that's expired from your medication counter. Once you're done with your dosage for the prescription medication, make sure you follow all the instructions for the disposal that have been indicated on the label. Avoid flushing the medication down the toilet unless the instructions advise you to do so.

If the accident victim is a woman, there are certain things to consider when getting prescription medication. You should let your doctor know:

- If you're trying to get pregnant or if you already are. Some drugs are harmful to an unborn baby, and if you've been trying, some medications can hinder the process. If there's a possibility that you might be pregnant, ensure you ask as many questions as possible about the potential side effects of the drugs you're being given to the fetus.

- In case you're a nursing mother, you should make it a point to ask the physician if any medication you're taking to heal from a domestic home accident is safe for the baby. Drugs are often secreted into the milk when the baby breastfeeds.

- In case you're taking birth control pills, some of the prescription drugs that you take for your accident might make the birth control pills ineffective. So while you're at the doctor's office, be sure to ask about this possibility so that you do not end up with an unplanned pregnancy.

- Some prescription drugs affect fertility. As such, it's worth asking questions regarding fertility so that you do not end up suffering this consequence in case you were trying to have a baby.

Some Questions to Ask About Side Effects
- Will there be any side effects to the medication?

- Are there side effects that should make you stop taking the medication immediately?

- Should you call the pharmacist or the doctor immediately if there are side effects or should this be done only if the side effects persist?

- Should, the victim, seek further treatment for the accident in case the side effects do not stop soon?

- How quickly will the medication work?

Chapter 19

Other Options for Treatment and Healing from Domestic Accidents

Massage Therapy

Through massage therapy, the soft tissues in your body are manipulated through certain massage techniques that require the use of the hands, elbows, fingers, the feet, or even a device. Therapeutic massages relieve the pain that a domestic accident victim may be experiencing by relaxing any painful tendons, muscles, and joints. Through massage therapy, you can also help relieve some of the stress and anxiety that came with the accident.

Physiotherapy

Physiotherapy as a treatment method is all about restoring, maintaining, and making the most of the ability of a patient to move or function properly, especially if they have sustained injuries from domestic accidents like falls. It works effectively through physical rehabilitation, prevention of further injuries, health, and fitness. Through physiotherapy, the accident victim is involved in their treatment. They have to maintain a level of discipline so that they heal completely. Physiotherapy is helpful for the following:

- Pain in the neck or back that's a result of issues in the skeleton or the victim's muscles

- Problems within one's bones, muscles, joints, and ligaments as a result of a domestic accident

- It helps alleviate fatigue and depression as a result of the accident

- It helps stiffness, swelling, and loss of muscle strength

Surgery

Some domestic accidents are more serious, and to heal from them, there is a need for surgery. Surgery involves cutting through the victim's body, abrading, or making changes in the victim's body so that they heal from the accident. It can be a major surgery or just a minor one depending on the extent of the injury.

Before the victim undergoes surgery, it's worth considering all the options. Meet the surgeon and get as much information as possible about the techniques that will be used and the pros and cons of each technique.

You should also rely on your connections to ensure a skilled and experienced medical team handles the case. Establish a good rapport with the doctor or the surgeon so that you have a great overall experience.

In case there is still a level of uncertainty within you, seek a second opinion. This will help you undergo the procedure with ease and recover much faster. Remember, your attitude towards recovery helps a great deal, and it needs to be positive from the start.

Conclusion

Unfortunately, accidents do happen in your home and while they might cause mild or severe pain, you need to know how to prevent future occurrences. You also need to know how to treat the accident victims quickly so that they do not develop further complications.

Should you go for home remedies to help heal from domestic accidents, don't forget to note that some of them have not been proven to work, while others might require some patience for you to see the results. OTC medication can be helpful, but you need to follow strict guidelines so that you do not make the situation worse.

Remember, the most important thing to do when one suffers an accident is to ensure they heal from it as fast as possible and that they heal completely. Providing fast, supportive action is the key. Do not shy away from a doctor's visit if there is any uncertainly. And if it's an emergency call 911.

Emergency Numbers to Keep on Hand

1. Poison Control Center

   1-800-822-1222

   or

   www.poison.org

   To add poison control as a contact in your phone, text POISON to 7979797.

2. Animal Poison Control Center (if your animal ingests poison)

   (888) 426-4435

3. Your family doctors

4. Local Electricity Company

5. Animal Control

6. Emergency contracts (friends, family, etc.)

7. Insurance agent

8. Emergency contacts for your children should you be unable to care for them

References

https://www.webmd.com/skin-problems-and-treatments/guide/bruises-article#1

https://www.mayoclinic.org/healthy-lifestyle/healthy-aging/in-depth/easy-bruising/art-20045762

https://ourstory.jnj.com/birth-first-aid-kit

https://www.medicalnewstoday.com/articles/321807#causes-of-strains

https://www.medicalnewstoday.com/articles/321807

https://www.medicinenet.com/sprained_ankle/article.htm

https://kidshealth.org/en/parents/safety-cuts.html

https://www.mayoclinic.org/diseases-conditions/burns/symptoms-causes/syc-20370539

https://familydoctor.org/burns-preventing-burns-in-your-home/

https://www.sharecare.com/health/first-aid-for-choking/what-common-causes-chiking-adult

https://nyulangone.org/conditions/poisoning-in-children/types

https://www.webmd.com/children/prevent-poisoning-home#1

https://kidshealth.org/en/parents/safety-poisoning.html

https://www.childrensmn.org/2016/03/24/8-tips-to-prevent-poisoning/

https://sharkclean.co.uk/7-common-household-accidents-avoid/

https://www.slhn.org/blog/2015/5-common-home-accidents-and-how-to-prevent-them

https://www.smrtindiana.com/blog/2014/3/31/5-reasons-why-first-aid-training-is-important

https://www.achievefirstaid.com/types-of-first-aid/

https://www.emergencyfirstresponse.com/5-reasons-why-basic-first-aid-knowledge-is-essential/

https://my.clevelandclinic.org/health/diseases/12063-burns

https://www.webmd.com/pain-management/qa/what-are-the-symptoms-of-burns

https://www.healthline.com/health/near-drowning#symptoms

https://www.healthline.com/health/dry-drowning

https://www.nhs.uk/conditions/poisoning/symptoms/

https://www.mayoclinic.org/first-aid/first-aid-choking/basics/art-20056637

https://kidshealth.org/en/parents/falls-sheet.html

https://www.mayoclinic.org/first-aid/first-aid-poisoning/basics/art-20056657

https://www.medicalnewstoday.com/articles/325260#medications

https://food.ndtv.com/health/7-effective-home-remedies-to-heal-open-wounds-1817835

https://food.ndtv.com/food-drinks/5-effective-home-remedies-for-mild-burns-1762840

https://www.readersdigest.ca/health/conditions/home-remedies-for-burns/

https://www.medicalnewstoday.com/articles/319768#remedies-to-avoid

https://electronichealthreporter.com/most-effective-home-remedies-to-recover-from-a-sprained-ankle/

https://www.sochealth.co.uk/2016/12/27/greatest-advantages-using-natural-remedies/

https://www.dummies.com/health/the-benefits-of-natural-medicine/

http://www.stauros.org/factors-to-consider-when-purchasing-over-the-counter-drugs/

https://www.policygenius.com/blog/how-to-stay-under-your-budget-for-over-the-counter-drugs/

https://www.emergencyphysicians.org/article/doc-blog/when---and-when-not---to-call-an-ambulance

https://www.webmd.com/mental-health/addiction/abuse-of-prescription-drugs#1

https://www.healthywomen.org/your-care/medication-safety

https://www.collegept.org/patients/what-is-physiotherapy

www.ingramcontent.com/pod-product-compliance
Lightning Source LLC
Chambersburg PA
CBHW062110020426
42335CB00013B/907